CONTENTS

THE COOKBOOK FOR DIABETICS

100 Dishes From Around The World

Dr Bhaskar Bora

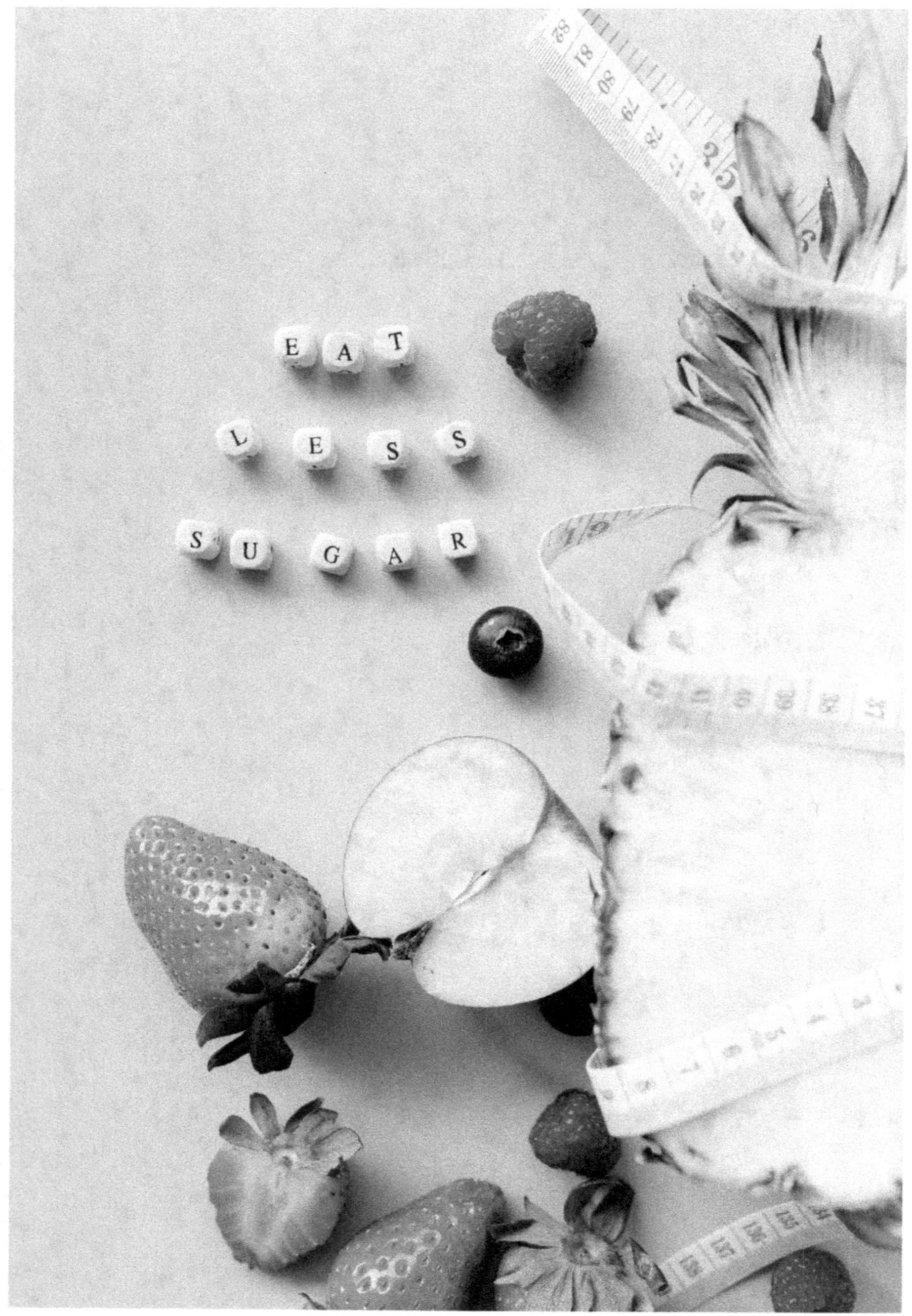
EAT
LESS
SUGAR

A PERSONAL NOTE FROM THE AUTHOR

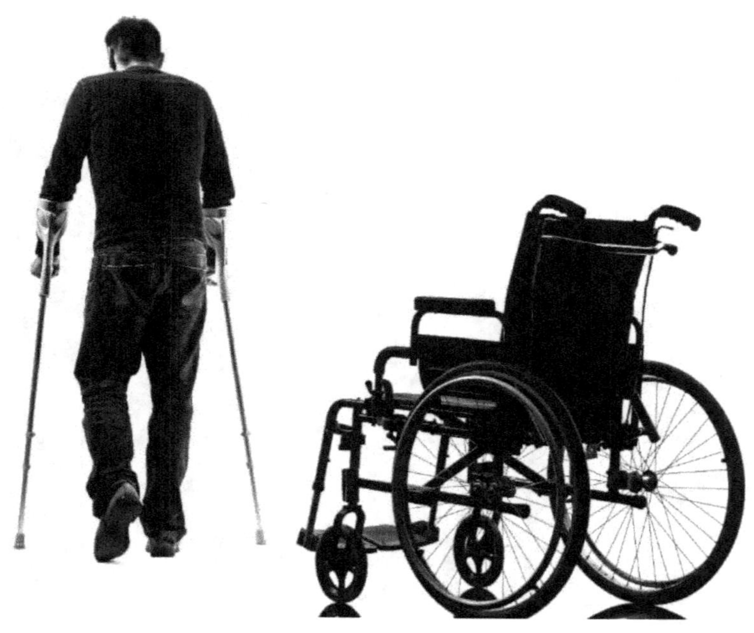

Though laden with unexpected trials and hardships, my journey has blossomed into a story of profound transformation—a journey that has led me to discover purpose, not in the towering milestones of success, but in the quiet, tender moments of love, care, and presence. What you hold in your hands is not merely a collection of recipes, but a testament to resilience—a narrative stitched together with threads of struggle, acceptance, and, in time, renewal.

There was a time when the story of my life played out with certainty and clarity, like a symphony where each note was perfectly placed. As a Doctor, my days were woven with the pulse of life itself—healing, comforting, offering hope where none had been. I wore my white coat with pride, for it was not just a garment but a symbol of who I was. The work I did, and the lives I touched, gave meaning to my every breath. My identity was fused with my role as a healer as if I had been born to follow that path.

But life, with its intricate unpredictability, had other plans. In a single, unforeseen moment, the world I had so carefully built was undone—first with a spinal cord injury that took away the physical strength I had always known, and then with the looming shadow of cancer, a reminder of how fragile life truly is. The vibrant world of medicine, where I once found purpose and joy, suddenly slipped beyond my reach. What once was filled with meaning became a void, vast and silent, leaving me to ask the questions I never thought I would need to face.

The bustling hospital hallways were exchanged for the quiet solitude of my home, where I was no longer a "Doctor." My hands, once steady with the knowledge of healing, trembled in the face of an unknown future. Who was I without the title, the purpose, and the work that defined me? I stood at the edge of this new reality, uncertain and untethered, wondering what life could offer beyond what I had known.

In the silence of that transition, I discovered something unexpected. What once seemed like an unfamiliar, distant role —being a disabled husband and a disabled father—became the essence of my existence. And within that shift, I found cooking. What began as an effort to nurture my family soon became a source of healing for me. In the rhythm of chopping, stirring, and tasting, I discovered a new purpose. Cooking became a language through which I reconnected with life, a practice that grounded me when everything else felt adrift and connected to the ones I love.

These past few years spent creating nourishing, simple meals, have been my lifeline—a daily practice of care for the people I love and for myself. Exploring different cuisines, experimenting with flavours, reading about ingredients and techniques—all of it became not just a pastime but a pathway to reclaiming my identity. Through cooking, I found a way forward, one meal at a time.

What I share with you now through this book, and those that will follow, are the lessons learned along the way. They are simple, practical, and grounded in love. These recipes and cooking tips are not adorned with glossy images or extravagant flourishes, but they carry with them the essence of resilience, creativity, and joy. I hope that they bring as much warmth and nourishment to your home as they have to mine, and that in their simplicity, you find a way to savour the moments spent with the ones you cherish.

We cannot control what the universe throws at us, but how we react to those curveballs defines who we are and what we make of our lives.

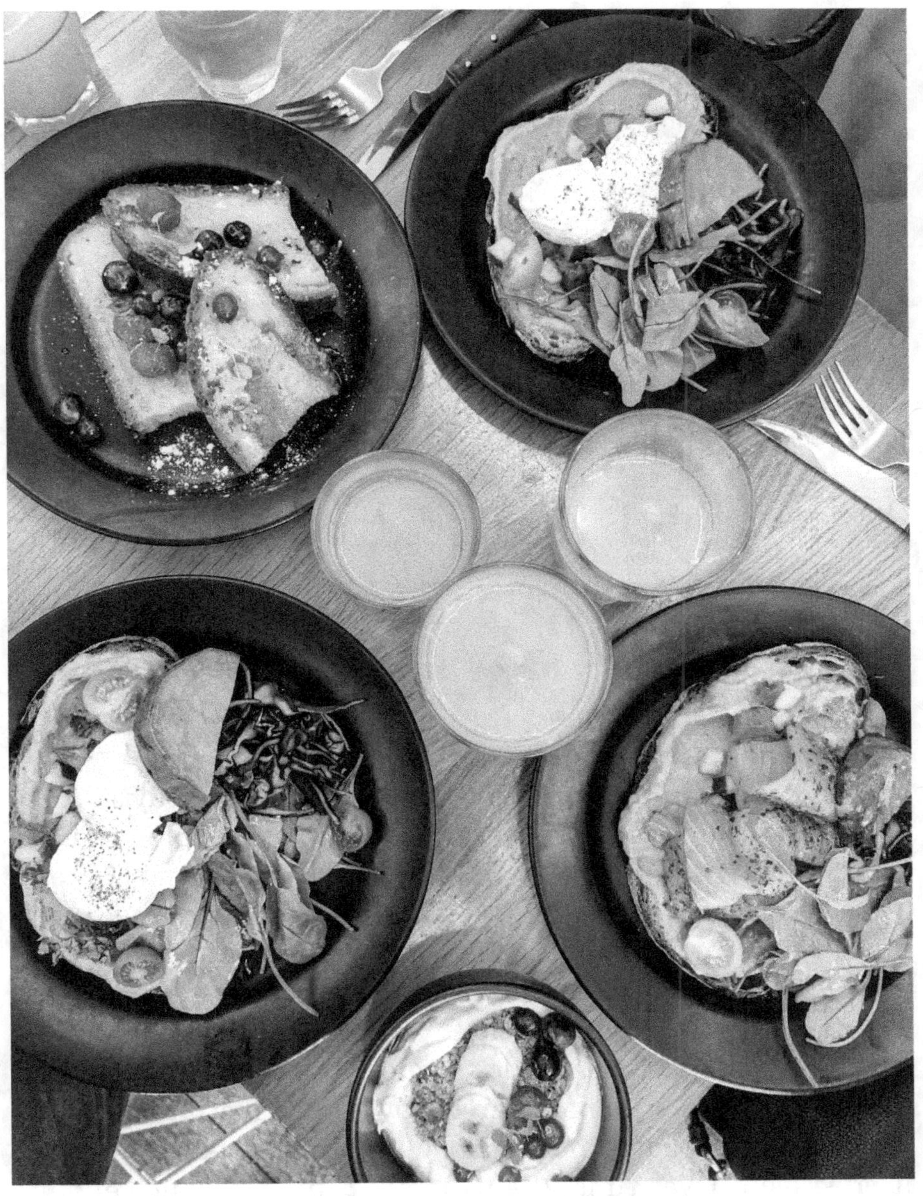

CHAPTER 1: INTRODUCTION TO COOKING FOR PEOPLE WITH DIABETES

Understanding Diabetes And Nutrition

History and Overview:
Diabetes is a chronic condition that impairs the body's ability to process blood glucose, otherwise known as blood sugar. There are two main types of diabetes: Type 1 and Type 2. Type 1 diabetes, often diagnosed in children and young adults, is an autoimmune condition where the body attacks insulin-producing cells in the pancreas. Without insulin, glucose from the food we eat cannot enter the cells and be used for energy. Type 2 diabetes, which is more prevalent and typically develops in adults, is characterized by insulin resistance. In this condition, the body produces insulin, but the cells do not use it effectively. Over time, the pancreas cannot produce enough insulin to maintain normal blood glucose levels.

Importance of Diet in Managing Diabetes:
Diet plays a crucial role in managing diabetes. Consuming a balanced diet helps maintain steady blood glucose levels,

reduces the risk of diabetes-related complications, and improves overall health. Key dietary goals include:
- Carbohydrate Management: Focus on complex carbohydrates with a low glycaemic index such as whole grains, vegetables, and legumes. These carbohydrates break down more slowly, preventing rapid spikes in blood sugar.
- Protein: Incorporate lean protein sources like poultry, fish, beans, and legumes. Protein helps stabilize blood sugar levels and promotes satiety.
- Healthy Fats: Include healthy fats from sources like avocados, nuts, seeds, and olive oil. These fats support heart health and provide essential fatty acids.
- Fiber: A high-fibre diet can help manage blood sugar levels and improve digestive health. Foods high in fibre include vegetables, fruits, whole grains, and legumes.
- Vitamins and Minerals: Ensure adequate intake of essential vitamins and minerals to support overall health and prevent deficiencies that can exacerbate diabetic complications.

Monitoring and Portion Control:
For individuals with diabetes, monitoring blood glucose levels and being mindful of portion sizes are critical. Regular monitoring helps understand how different foods affect blood sugar levels, allowing for better dietary choices. Portion control prevents overeating, which can lead to weight gain and increased blood glucose levels.

"Let food be thy medicine and medicine be thy food."
– Hippocrates

Planning a Diabetic-Friendly Diet

Meal Planning Basics:
Planning meals ahead of time is a fundamental strategy

for managing diabetes. A well-thought-out meal plan helps maintain consistent blood sugar levels and prevents last-minute unhealthy food choices. Here are some tips for creating a diabetic-friendly meal plan:

- Balance Macronutrients: Ensure each meal contains a balanced mix of carbohydrates, proteins, and fats. This balance helps control blood sugar levels and provides sustained energy.
- Focus on Whole Foods: Prioritize whole, unprocessed foods. These foods are naturally rich in nutrients and free from added sugars and unhealthy fats.
- Regular Eating Schedule: Establish regular meal and snack times to keep blood sugar levels stable throughout the day. Skipping meals can lead to significant fluctuations in blood glucose levels.
- Hydration: Staying well-hydrated is important for everyone, especially those with diabetes. Water is the best choice, but herbal teas and infused waters can add variety.

Grocery Shopping Tips:
Smart grocery shopping is the first step towards preparing healthy meals. Here are some tips for shopping with diabetes in mind:
- Shop the Perimeter: Focus on the outer aisles of the grocery store where fresh produce, lean meats, and dairy products are typically located. These areas are usually stocked with whole, unprocessed foods.
- Read Labels: Become familiar with reading food labels to check for hidden sugars, unhealthy fats, and other undesirable ingredients. Look for foods with high fibre content and minimal added sugars.
- Stock Up on Staples: Keep a supply of diabetic-friendly staples like whole grains (brown rice, quinoa, whole wheat pasta), legumes (lentils, chickpeas, black beans), and fresh vegetables (spinach, broccoli, bell peppers).

Example of a Daily Meal Plan:

Here's an example of a balanced daily meal plan for someone managing diabetes:
- Breakfast: Greek yogurt with berries and nuts. This meal provides protein, healthy fats, and fibre.
- Lunch: Grilled chicken salad with mixed greens, cherry tomatoes, cucumber, and a light vinaigrette. This meal offers lean protein, fresh vegetables, and healthy fats.
- Snack: An apple with a handful of almonds. This snack is rich in fibre and healthy fats.
- Dinner: Quinoa salad with chickpeas, roasted vegetables, and a lemon-tahini dressing. This meal is high in fibre, protein, and healthy fats.
- Dessert: A small portion of dark chocolate with a few strawberries. This treat satisfies sweet cravings without causing a spike in blood sugar levels.

"To eat is a necessity, but to eat intelligently is an art

– François de La Rochefoucauld

Cooking Techniques for Diabetics

Healthy Cooking Methods:
Choosing the right cooking methods can significantly impact the nutritional quality of meals. Here are some healthy cooking techniques:
- Grilling: Grilling meats and vegetables enhances flavour without the need for added fats. Use a grill or grill pan to cook lean meats, fish, and a variety of vegetables.
- Baking: Baking is a versatile and healthy cooking method. Use it to prepare everything from baked chicken and fish to roasted vegetables and whole-grain casseroles.

- Steaming: Steaming preserves nutrients and enhances the natural flavours of foods. Steam vegetables, fish, and even some grains for a light and healthy meal.
- Stir-Frying: This quick cooking method uses high heat and minimal oil. Stir-fry a mix of vegetables, lean proteins, and whole grains for a nutritious meal.

Reducing Sugar and Salt:
Cutting back on sugar and salt is essential for managing diabetes. Here are some tips to help:
- Use Natural Sweeteners: Substitute refined sugar with natural sweeteners like stevia, monk fruit, or small amounts of honey. These alternatives have a lower glycaemic index and less impact on blood sugar levels.
- Flavour with Herbs and Spices: Enhance the taste of dishes with a variety of herbs and spices. Experiment with basil, cilantro, dill, oregano, thyme, cinnamon, nutmeg, and turmeric to add flavour without relying on salt.
- Read Labels: Be aware of hidden sugars and sodium in processed foods. Opt for low-sodium and no-added-sugar versions when possible.

Preparing Balanced Meals:
A balanced meal includes a mix of carbohydrates, proteins, and fats. Here are some ideas for balanced meals:
- Breakfast: A veggie omelette made with egg whites, spinach, tomatoes, and a sprinkle of cheese. Serve with a slice of whole-grain toast.
- Lunch: A quinoa and chickpea salad with mixed greens, cucumbers, and a lemon vinaigrette.
- Dinner: Grilled salmon with a side of steamed broccoli and roasted sweet potatoes.

"One cannot think well, love well, sleep well, if one has not dined well."

– Virginia Woolf

Delicious and Diabetic-Friendly Recipes

Breakfast Ideas:
Starting the day with a nutritious breakfast can help stabilize blood sugar levels and provide energy. Here are some ideas:
- Greek Yogurt with Berries and Nuts: Greek yogurt is high in protein and low in carbohydrates. Topping it with fresh berries and a sprinkle of nuts adds fibre and healthy fats, making it a balanced and satisfying meal.
- Oatmeal with Chia Seeds and Berries: Oatmeal is a whole grain that digests slowly, providing sustained energy. Adding chia seeds boosts the fibre content, and berries add natural sweetness and antioxidants.
- Veggie Omelette: An omelette made with egg whites or a mix of whole eggs and egg whites, filled with sautéed spinach, tomatoes, and mushrooms, provides a low-carb, high-protein start to the day.

Lunch and Dinner Options:
Balanced meals for lunch and dinner are essential for managing blood sugar levels throughout the day. Here are some suggestions:
- Quinoa Salad with Chickpeas and Veggies: Quinoa is a whole grain that is high in protein and fibre. Combining it with chickpeas and a variety of fresh vegetables creates a filling and nutritious meal. A light lemon-tahini dressing adds flavour without unnecessary calories.
- Grilled Chicken Salad: Lean protein from grilled chicken paired with mixed greens, cherry tomatoes, cucumber, and a light vinaigrette makes for a refreshing and healthy meal. Add avocado for healthy fats and extra flavour.
- Vegetable Stir-Fry with Tofu: Tofu is a great source of plant-based protein. Stir-frying it with a mix of colourful vegetables

like bell peppers, broccoli, and snap peas in a light soy sauce or tamari creates a quick and nutrient-dense meal.

Snack Ideas:
Healthy snacks help prevent blood sugar spikes and keep hunger at bay. Here are some options:
- Apple Slices with Almond Butter: Apples are high in fibre and provide a natural sweetness. Pairing them with almond butter adds protein and healthy fats.
- Hummus with Veggie Sticks: Hummus made from chickpeas is a good source of protein and fibre. Serve it with a variety of veggie sticks like carrots, celery, and bell peppers.
- Mixed Nuts and Seeds: A handful of mixed nuts and seeds provides a good mix of protein, healthy fats, and fibre, making it a satisfying and portable snack.

"Cooking is at once child's play and adult joy. And cooking done with care is an act of love."

– Craig Claiborne

Tips for Dining Out and Managing Cravings

Dining Out Tips:
Eating out can be challenging for diabetics, but with careful choices, it can be enjoyable and healthy. Here are some tips:
- Research Menus: Look up the menu online before going to the restaurant to identify healthy options. Many restaurants offer nutritional information that can help you make informed choices.
- Ask for Modifications: Don't hesitate to ask for modifications to make dishes healthier. Request grilled instead of fried, ask for dressings and sauces on the side, and substitute vegetables for

starchy sides.

- Portion Control: Restaurant portions are often larger than necessary. Consider sharing a meal with a dining companion or asking for a to-go box when the meal arrives and setting aside half for later.
- Choose Wisely: Opt for lean proteins like grilled chicken or fish and fill your plate with non-starchy vegetables. Avoid dishes that are breaded, fried, or smothered in heavy sauces.

Managing Cravings:

Cravings are natural, but they can be managed with some strategies:

- Healthy Snacks: Keep healthy snacks like nuts, seeds, fresh fruit, and vegetable sticks with hummus on hand to avoid reaching for unhealthy options.
- Stay Hydrated: Sometimes thirst is mistaken for hunger. Drink plenty of water throughout the day to stay hydrated and help control cravings.
- Mindful Eating: Pay attention to your hunger cues and eat slowly to enjoy your food and recognize when you're full. Mindful eating can prevent overeating and help you make better food choices.
- Healthy Alternatives: Find healthy alternatives to your favourite treats. For example, if you crave sweets, try a piece of dark chocolate or a fruit-based dessert. If you crave something salty, opt for air-popped popcorn or roasted chickpeas.

Building a Support System:

Managing diabetes can be challenging, but having a support system can make a big difference. Surround yourself with friends and family who understand your dietary needs and can offer encouragement and support. Consider joining a support group for people with diabetes, either in person or online, to share experiences and get tips from others who are managing the condition.

"Your diet is a bank account. Good food choices are good investments."

– Bethenny Frankel

CHAPTER 2: HEALTHY COOKING CAN BE EASY, TASTY, AFFORDABLE, AND FUN-FILLED

The Fundamentals Of Healthy Cooking

Introduction to Healthy Cooking:
Healthy cooking does not mean sacrificing flavour, convenience, or budget. With the right strategies and mindset, you can create meals that are not only nutritious but also delicious, quick to prepare, affordable, and enjoyable to make.

Balancing Nutrition and Flavour:
A common misconception is that healthy food is bland or boring. However, using fresh ingredients, herbs, and spices can enhance the flavours of your dishes while keeping them nutritious. Here are some fundamentals:
- Use Fresh Ingredients: Fresh vegetables, fruits, lean meats, and whole grains are the building blocks of healthy meals.
- Incorporate Herbs and Spices: Herbs and spices can add depth and flavour without the need for excessive salt or sugar. Experiment with basil, cilantro, thyme, cumin, paprika, and

other seasonings.
- Healthy Fats: Incorporate healthy fats like olive oil, avocado, nuts, and seeds to add richness and improve nutrient absorption.

Meal Prep Basics:
Meal prepping can make healthy eating more convenient and less time-consuming. By preparing ingredients or complete meals in advance, you can save time during the week and ensure you always have healthy options available.
- Batch Cooking: Cook large batches of staples like grains, beans, and proteins that can be used in various meals throughout the week.
- Chop Ahead: Pre-chop vegetables and store them in airtight containers to make cooking faster.
- Freezer-Friendly Meals: Prepare and freeze meals like soups, stews, and casseroles that can be easily reheated.

"Good food is the foundation of genuine happiness."

– Auguste Escoffier

Making Healthy Cooking Easy and Time-Saving

Quick and Simple Recipes:
Healthy cooking doesn't have to be complicated. Here are some tips for keeping it simple:
- One-Pot Meals: Reduce cleanup time by making one-pot meals like stir-fries, soups, and stews.
- Sheet Pan Dinners: Roast vegetables and proteins together on a single sheet pan for a quick and easy dinner.
- Salads and Wraps: Prepare hearty salads and wraps with a variety of fresh ingredients for quick, no-cook meals.

Kitchen Tools and Gadgets:
Using the right tools can make cooking more efficient and

enjoyable. Consider investing in these gadgets:
- Slow Cooker/Instant Pot: These appliances can help you prepare meals with minimal effort. Just add ingredients, set the timer, and let it cook.
- Blender/Food Processor: Perfect for making smoothies, soups, sauces, and dips quickly.
- Sharp Knives and Cutting Boards: Good quality knives make chopping and prepping faster and safer.

Planning Ahead:
Effective meal planning saves time and reduces stress. Here are some strategies:
- Weekly Menu: Plan your meals for the week and make a shopping list based on the menu.
- Prep Days: Dedicate a day or two each week to meal prep. This can include cooking grains, roasting vegetables, and portioning snacks.
- Double Recipes: Cook double batches of recipes so you can enjoy leftovers or freeze portions for later.

"The secret of success in life is to eat what you like and let the food fight it out inside."

– Mark Twain

Affordable Healthy Cooking

Budget-Friendly Tips:
Eating healthy doesn't have to be expensive. Here are some ways to keep costs down:
- Buy in Bulk: Purchase staples like grains, beans, and nuts in bulk to save money.
- Seasonal Produce: Buy fruits and vegetables that are in season. They are often cheaper and fresher.
- Frozen and Canned Goods: Frozen and canned fruits and

vegetables can be just as nutritious as fresh ones and are often more affordable and long-lasting.
- Reduce Meat Consumption: Incorporate more plant-based meals into your diet. Beans, lentils, and tofu are cost-effective protein sources.

Smart Shopping:
Making thoughtful choices at the grocery store can help you stay within your budget:
- Plan Your Meals: Create a meal plan and shopping list before heading to the store to avoid impulse purchases.
- Compare Prices: Check unit prices to find the best deals and consider store brands, which are often cheaper.
- Use Coupons and Sales: Take advantage of sales, discounts, and coupons to save money on healthy foods.

Cooking at Home:
Preparing meals at home is generally more affordable than eating out. Here's how to make the most of home cooking:
- Cook from Scratch: Processed and pre-packaged foods can be more expensive and less nutritious. Cooking from scratch allows you to control ingredients and costs.
- Repurpose Leftovers: Use leftovers creatively to make new meals. For example, roast chicken can be used in salads, soups, and wraps.
- Minimize Waste: Store food properly to extend its shelf life and reduce waste. Use every part of ingredients where possible, such as vegetable peels for broth.

> *"A recipe has no soul. You, as the cook, must bring soul to the recipe." – Thomas Keller*

Making Healthy Cooking Tasty

Flavour Boosters:

Enhance the flavour of your dishes with these tips:
- Herbs and Spices: Fresh herbs like basil, cilantro, and parsley, and dried spices like cumin, coriander, and paprika can elevate the taste of any dish.
- Citrus: Lemon and lime juice can add brightness and acidity, balancing flavours and reducing the need for salt.
- Healthy Sauces and Dressings: Create homemade sauces and dressings using yogurt, avocado, mustard, and vinegars. These can add a burst of flavour without unhealthy additives.

Experimenting with Recipes:
Don't be afraid to try new recipes and ingredients:
- Cultural Cuisines: Explore different cuisines like Mediterranean, Asian, or Middle Eastern for diverse and flavourful dishes.
- Ingredient Swaps: Experiment with healthy ingredient swaps, like using Greek yogurt instead of sour cream or avocado instead of butter in baking.
- Cookbooks and Online Resources: Use cookbooks and online resources for inspiration and new ideas. There are countless healthy recipes available to suit every taste and dietary preference.

Cooking Techniques for Flavour:
Certain cooking techniques can enhance the natural flavours of foods:
- Roasting: Roasting vegetables and proteins brings out their natural sweetness and creates a delicious, caramelized flavour.
- Grilling: Grilling adds a smoky flavour to meats, fish, and vegetables, making them more appealing.
- Marinating: Marinating proteins and vegetables infuses them with flavour and can tenderize meats.

"People who love to eat are always the best people."

– Julia Child

Making Healthy Cooking Fun and Enjoyable

Cooking as a Social Activity:
Cooking can be a fun social activity to share with family and friends:
- Cooking Parties: Host a cooking party where everyone can participate in preparing a healthy meal. It's a great way to bond and share cooking tips.
- Family Involvement: Get the whole family involved in meal prep. Kids can help with washing vegetables, measuring ingredients, and setting the table.
- Cooking Classes: Consider taking a cooking class to learn new skills and recipes while meeting new people who share your interest in healthy eating.

Creative Presentation:
Make your meals visually appealing:
- Colourful Plates: Use a variety of colourful vegetables and fruits to make your dishes more vibrant and appetizing.
- Garnishes: Add fresh herbs, seeds, or a drizzle of healthy sauce as garnishes to elevate the presentation of your meals.
- Table Setting: Create a pleasant dining environment with a nicely set table, good lighting, and relaxing music.

Experimenting and Learning:
Embrace the learning process and have fun with it:
- Try New Recipes: Regularly try new recipes to keep things interesting. Challenge yourself to cook a new dish each week.
- Food Challenges: Set fun food challenges for yourself, like using only seasonal ingredients or cooking a meal with a specific theme.
- Document Your Journey: Keep a food diary or blog to document your cooking journey, share recipes, and reflect on what you've learned.

Enjoying the Process:
Cooking should be a pleasurable activity, not a chore:
- Mindful Cooking: Focus on the process of cooking, enjoying the smells, textures, and colors of the ingredients. This mindfulness can enhance your overall experience.
- Reward Yourself: Reward your efforts by taking the time to savour and enjoy the meals you've prepared. Share them with loved ones and appreciate the nourishment and joy they bring.

"Cooking is like love. It should be entered into with abandon or not at all." – Harriet Van Horne

GLOSSARY OF TERMS

Almond Flour: A type of flour made from finely ground almonds. It is commonly used in gluten-free and low-carb baking due to its high protein and low carbohydrate content.

Avocado: A fruit known for its high content of healthy fats, particularly monounsaturated fat. It is often used in salads, smoothies, and as a spread.

Baking: A cooking method that uses dry heat, typically in an oven, to cook food. Common baking foods include bread, cakes, pastries, and casseroles.

Batch Cooking: The process of preparing large quantities of food at once to be portioned out and stored for future meals, saving time and effort during the week.

Basil: A fragrant herb commonly used in Italian cuisine. It pairs well with tomatoes, garlic, and olive oil.

Blender: A kitchen appliance used to mix, puree, or emulsify food and other substances. Ideal for making smoothies, soups, and sauces.

Broccoli: A cruciferous vegetable rich in vitamins, minerals, and fibre. It can be eaten raw or cooked and is known for its numerous health benefits.

Brown Rice: A whole grain rice with the bran and germ intact, making it higher in fibre and nutrients compared to white rice.

Cauliflower: A versatile vegetable that can be used as a low-carb substitute for grains and legumes in recipes like rice, pizza crusts, and mashed potatoes.

Chia Seeds: Small black seeds from the Salvia hispanica plant. They are rich in omega-3 fatty acids, fibre, and protein, and are often used in puddings, smoothies, and baked goods.

Chickpeas: Also known as garbanzo beans, these legumes are high in protein and fibre. They are commonly used in salads, stews, and as the base for hummus.

Coconut Oil: An edible oil extracted from the kernel of mature coconuts. It is high in saturated fats and is often used in cooking and baking.

Complex Carbohydrates: Carbohydrates that are composed of longer chains of sugar molecules, such as those found in whole grains, vegetables, and legumes. They are digested more slowly and provide sustained energy.

Cumin: A spice made from the dried seeds of the Cuminum cyminum plant. It is commonly used in Middle Eastern, Indian, and Mexican cuisines.

Curry Powder: A blend of spices, typically including turmeric, coriander, cumin, and fenugreek. It is used to flavour dishes in Indian and Southeast Asian cuisines.

Dietary Fiber: A type of carbohydrate that the body cannot digest. It is found in plant foods such as fruits, vegetables, grains, and legumes, and helps regulate the body's use of sugars.

Dried Herbs and Spices: Dehydrated herbs and spices that retain the flavour of fresh ones and are used to season and enhance the taste of food.

Feta Cheese: A brined white cheese made from sheep's milk or a mixture of sheep and goat's milk. It is known for its crumbly texture and tangy flavour.

Fiber: A type of carbohydrate that the body cannot digest. It is essential for digestive health and helps regulate blood sugar levels.

Garlic: A plant in the onion family used for its pungent flavour in cooking and its health benefits. It is commonly used in a variety of cuisines worldwide.

Glycaemic Index: A measure of how quickly a food causes blood sugar levels to rise. Foods with a low glycaemic index are digested more slowly and have a less immediate impact on blood sugar levels.

Grains: Edible seeds from cereal crops such as wheat, rice, oats, and barley. Whole grains contain the entire grain kernel and are higher in nutrients and fibre compared to refined grains.

Grilling: A cooking method that involves dry heat applied to the surface of food, commonly from above or below. It imparts a smoky flavour and is often used for meats and vegetables.

Healthy Fats: Fats that are beneficial to health, including monounsaturated and polyunsaturated fats found in foods like avocados, nuts, seeds, and fish.

Herbs: Plants or plant parts used for their flavour, aroma, or medicinal properties. Common culinary herbs include basil, thyme, rosemary, and cilantro.

Instant Pot: A brand of multi-cooker that combines several cooking functions in one appliance, including pressure cooking, slow cooking, rice cooking, steaming, and sautéing.

Insulin: A hormone produced by the pancreas that regulates blood sugar levels by facilitating the uptake of glucose into cells.

Kale: A leafy green vegetable rich in vitamins A, C, and K. It is often used in salads, smoothies, and as a cooked green.

Lentils: Small legumes that come in various colors, including green, brown, and red. They are high in protein and fibre and are used in soups, stews, and salads.

Low-Carb: A dietary approach that limits the intake of carbohydrates, typically focusing on foods high in protein and fat, such as meats, fish, eggs, vegetables, and healthy fats.

Marinating: The process of soaking foods in a seasoned liquid mixture before cooking to add flavour and tenderize the meat.

Meal Prep: The practice of preparing meals and ingredients in advance to save time and ensure healthy eating throughout the week.

Monounsaturated Fats: A type of healthy fat found in olive oil, avocados, and certain nuts. These fats are beneficial for heart health.

Oats: A whole grain that is commonly eaten as oatmeal or used in baked goods. Oats are high in fibre and have numerous health benefits.

Olive Oil: An oil extracted from olives, commonly used in cooking, salad dressings, and as a dipping oil. It is high in monounsaturated fats and antioxidants.

Omelette: A dish made from beaten eggs cooked with butter or oil in a frying pan. It can be filled with various ingredients such as cheese, vegetables, and meats.

Pantry Staples: Basic ingredients that are commonly kept on hand in a pantry, such as grains, beans, spices, oils, and canned goods.

Parsley: A bright green, biennial herb used as a garnish and in cooking for its fresh flavour. It is rich in vitamins and antioxidants.

Plant-Based: A diet that emphasizes foods derived from plants, including vegetables, fruits, nuts, seeds, oils, whole grains, and legumes, with few or no animal products.

Portion Control: Managing the amount of food consumed in one sitting to avoid overeating and maintain a balanced diet.

Protein: A macronutrient essential for building and repairing tissues, making enzymes, and supporting overall health. Sources include meat, fish, beans, and nuts.

Quinoa: A gluten-free grain that is high in protein and fibre. It is often used as a substitute for rice or couscous.

Refined Sugars: Sugars that have been processed and stripped of their natural nutrients, commonly found in sweets, baked goods, and processed foods.

Roasting: A dry heat cooking method where food is cooked in an oven, typically resulting in a caramelized exterior and tender interior.

Salmon: A type of fatty fish rich in omega-3 fatty acids, protein, and vitamins. It is commonly grilled, baked, or poached.

Sautéing: A cooking method that uses a small amount of oil or fat in a shallow pan over relatively high heat to cook food quickly.

Slow Cooker: A countertop electrical appliance used to cook foods slowly at a low temperature. It is ideal for making stews, soups, and other slow-cooked dishes.

Smoothie: A blended beverage typically made from fruits, vegetables, yogurt, and other nutritious ingredients. Smoothies can be a quick and healthy meal or snack.

Spinach: A leafy green vegetable that is high in iron, vitamins, and minerals. It can be eaten raw in salads or cooked in a variety of dishes.

Stir-Frying: A cooking method where ingredients are quickly fried in a small amount of oil over high heat while being stirred continuously.

Tahini: A paste made from ground sesame seeds, commonly used in Middle Eastern cuisine. It is an ingredient in hummus and other dishes.

Thyme: A fragrant herb used in cooking for its strong, earthy flavour. It pairs well with meats, vegetables, and soups.

Tofu: A protein-rich food made from soybeans. It is often used in vegetarian and vegan dishes as a meat substitute.

Turmeric: A bright yellow spice derived from the turmeric root, commonly used in Indian cuisine and known for its anti-inflammatory properties.

Vegetable Broth: A savoury liquid made by simmering vegetables, herbs, and spices. It is used as a base for soups, stews, and sauces.

Whole Grains: Grains that contain the entire grain kernel, including the bran, germ, and endosperm. Examples include brown rice, quinoa, and whole wheat.

Yogurt: A dairy product made by fermenting milk with bacteria. It is high in protein and probiotics, beneficial for digestive health.

Chapter 3: Breakfast

"Eat breakfast like a king, lunch like a prince, and dinner like a pauper."

– Adelle Davis

1. GREEK YOGURT WITH BERRIES AND NUTS

History:
Greek yogurt, known for its thick consistency and rich flavour, has its roots in the Mediterranean region. It has been a staple in Greek cuisine for centuries and has gained popularity worldwide for its high protein content and probiotic benefits.

Ingredients:
- 1 cup Greek yogurt
- 1/2 cup mixed berries (blueberries, strawberries, raspberries)
- 1/4 cup mixed nuts (almonds, walnuts, pistachios)
- 1 tablespoon honey (optional)

Possible Substitutes:
- Plant-based yogurt for a dairy-free option
- Different fruits such as kiwi or banana
- Seeds like sunflower or pumpkin seeds instead of nuts

Method of Preparation:
1. Scoop Greek yogurt into a bowl.
2. Top with mixed berries and nuts.
3. Drizzle with honey if desired.
4. Serve immediately.

Nutritional Value (per serving):
- Calories: 300

- Carbohydrates: 25g
- Protein: 18g
- Fat: 15g
- Fiber: 5g

Cost per Serving:
Approximately $3.50

2. AVOCADO TOAST

History:
Avocado toast has become a trendy breakfast option, especially popularized by the health-conscious millennials. It originated in Australia and quickly spread across the globe due to its simplicity and nutritional benefits.

Ingredients:
- 2 slices whole grain bread
- 1 ripe avocado
- 1 tablespoon lemon juice
- Salt and pepper to taste
- Optional toppings: cherry tomatoes, radishes, arugula

Possible Substitutes:
- Gluten-free bread for a gluten-free option
- Hummus or mashed beans instead of avocado

Method of Preparation:
1. Toast the bread slices until golden brown.
2. Mash the avocado in a bowl with lemon juice, salt, and pepper.
3. Spread the avocado mixture on the toasted bread.
4. Add optional toppings if desired.
5. Serve immediately.

Nutritional Value (per serving):
- Calories: 350
- Carbohydrates: 40g
- Protein: 10g
- Fat: 20g
- Fiber: 10g

Cost per Serving:
Approximately $2.50

3. OATMEAL WITH CHIA SEEDS AND BERRIES

History:
Oatmeal has been a breakfast staple for centuries, known for its heart-healthy benefits and versatility. Chia seeds, native to Central America, add an extra nutritional punch with their high omega-3 and fibre content.

Ingredients:
- 1 cup rolled oats
- 2 cups almond milk
- 1 tablespoon chia seeds
- 1/2 cup mixed berries
- 1 tablespoon honey or maple syrup (optional)

Possible Substitutes:
- Different plant-based milk options
- Other fruits like apples or bananas

Method of Preparation:
1. Combine oats and almond milk in a saucepan.
2. Cook over medium heat, stirring occasionally, until the oats are soft (about 5-7 minutes).
3. Stir in chia seeds and cook for another 2 minutes.
4. Serve topped with mixed berries and a drizzle of honey or maple syrup if desired.

Nutritional Value (per serving):
- Calories: 350
- Carbohydrates: 55g
- Protein: 10g
- Fat: 10g
- Fiber: 10g

Cost per Serving:
Approximately $2.00

4. SCRAMBLED EGGS WITH SPINACH AND TOMATOES

History:
Scrambled eggs are a breakfast classic found in many cultures. Adding spinach and tomatoes not only enhances the flavour but also boosts the nutritional value, making it a well-rounded meal.

Ingredients:
- 3 eggs
- 1/2 cup fresh spinach, chopped
- 1/4 cup cherry tomatoes, halved
- 1 tablespoon olive oil
- Salt and pepper to taste

Possible Substitutes:
- Egg whites for a lower cholesterol option
- Other greens like kale or Swiss chard

Method of Preparation:
1. Heat olive oil in a non-stick skillet over medium heat.
2. Add spinach and tomatoes, cooking until spinach is wilted.
3. Beat the eggs in a bowl, then pour into the skillet.
4. Cook, stirring frequently, until eggs are scrambled and cooked through.
5. Season with salt and pepper to taste.
6. Serve immediately.

Nutritional Value (per serving):
- Calories: 250
- Carbohydrates: 5g
- Protein: 18g
- Fat: 18g
- Fiber: 2g

Cost per Serving:
Approximately $2.00

5. SMOOTHIE BOWL WITH KALE AND BANANAS

History:
Smoothie bowls have become a popular health trend, combining the convenience of smoothies with the texture and toppings of a bowl of cereal. They originated in health food circles and quickly gained popularity for their versatility and nutrition.

Ingredients:
- 1 cup kale leaves
- 1 banana
- 1/2 cup almond milk
- 1/2 cup mixed berries
- 1 tablespoon chia seeds
- 1 tablespoon nuts (optional)

Possible Substitutes:
- Spinach instead of kale
- Different fruits for variety

Method of Preparation:
1. Blend kale, banana, and almond milk until smooth.
2. Pour into a bowl and top with mixed berries, chia seeds, and nuts if desired.
3. Serve immediately.

Nutritional Value (per serving):

- Calories: 300
- Carbohydrates: 45g
- Protein: 8g
- Fat: 10g
- Fiber: 10g

Cost per Serving:
Approximately $3.00

"Breakfast is the most important meal of the day."

— Unknown

6. COTTAGE CHEESE WITH PINEAPPLE AND ALMONDS

History:
Cottage cheese has been a popular dairy product for centuries, known for its high protein content and versatility. Combining it with pineapple and almonds creates a balanced, refreshing breakfast option.

Ingredients:
- 1 cup cottage cheese
- 1/2 cup pineapple chunks
- 2 tablespoons sliced almonds
- 1 tablespoon honey (optional)

Possible Substitutes:
- Greek yogurt instead of cottage cheese
- Different fruits like peaches or berries

Method of Preparation:
1. Place cottage cheese in a bowl.
2. Top with pineapple chunks and sliced almonds.
3. Drizzle with honey if desired.
4. Serve immediately.

Nutritional Value (per serving):
- Calories: 250
- Carbohydrates: 20g

- Protein: 20g
- Fat: 10g
- Fiber: 2g

Cost per Serving:
Approximately $2.50

7. WHOLE WHEAT PANCAKES WITH BERRIES

History:
Pancakes have been enjoyed for centuries, with variations found in nearly every culture. Whole wheat pancakes provide a healthier alternative to traditional white flour pancakes, adding fibre and nutrients.

Ingredients:
- 1 cup whole wheat flour
- 1 tablespoon baking powder
- 1 cup almond milk
- 1 egg
- 1 tablespoon honey
- 1/2 cup mixed berries

Possible Substitutes:
- Gluten-free flour for a gluten-free option
- Different fruits for topping

Method of Preparation:
1. Mix whole wheat flour and baking powder in a bowl.
2. In another bowl, whisk together almond milk, egg, and honey.
3. Combine wet and dry ingredients, stirring until smooth.
4. Heat a non-stick skillet over medium heat and pour batter to form pancakes.

5. Cook until bubbles form on the surface, then flip and cook until golden brown.
6. Serve topped with mixed berries.

Nutritional Value (per serving):
- Calories: 300
- Carbohydrates: 45g
- Protein: 10g
- Fat: 8g
- Fiber: 6g

Cost per Serving:
Approximately $2.50

8. CHIA SEED PUDDING

History:
Chia seeds were a staple food of the ancient Aztecs and Mayans. Today, they are prized for their high fibre, omega-3 fatty acids, and protein content, making chia seed pudding a popular breakfast choice.

Ingredients:
- 1/4 cup chia seeds
- 1 cup almond milk
- 1 tablespoon honey or maple syrup
- 1/2 teaspoon vanilla extract
- Fresh fruit for topping

Possible Substitutes:
- Different plant-based milks
- Various sweeteners like stevia

Method of Preparation:
1. In a bowl, mix chia seeds, almond milk, honey, and vanilla extract.
2. Stir well and let sit for 5 minutes, then stir again to prevent clumping.
3. Cover and refrigerate for at least 2 hours or overnight.
4. Serve topped with fresh fruit.

Nutritional Value (per serving):
- Calories: 200

- Carbohydrates: 20g
- Protein: 5g
- Fat: 10g
- Fiber: 12g

Cost per Serving:
Approximately $1.50

9. VEGGIE OMELETTE

History:
The omelette has a long history, with variations found in French, Spanish, and American cuisines. Adding vegetables makes it a nutritious and balanced breakfast option.

Ingredients:
- 3 eggs
- 1

/4 cup bell peppers, chopped
- 1/4 cup onions, chopped
- 1/4 cup mushrooms, sliced
- 1 tablespoon olive oil
- Salt and pepper to taste

Possible Substitutes:
- Egg whites for lower cholesterol
- Any vegetables you prefer

Method of Preparation:
1. Heat olive oil in a non-stick skillet over medium heat.
2. Sauté bell peppers, onions, and mushrooms until tender.
3. Beat the eggs in a bowl, then pour over the vegetables.
4. Cook until the eggs are set, folding the omelette in half.
5. Season with salt and pepper to taste.
6. Serve immediately.

Nutritional Value (per serving):
- Calories: 250
- Carbohydrates: 5g

- Protein: 18g
- Fat: 18g
- Fiber: 2g

Cost per Serving:
Approximately $2.00

10. BUCKWHEAT PORRIDGE

History:
Buckwheat has been a staple in Eastern European cuisine for centuries. It's a nutritious, gluten-free grain that is rich in fibre and minerals, making it an excellent breakfast option.

Ingredients:
- 1 cup buckwheat groats
- 2 cups water
- 1 cup almond milk
- 1 tablespoon honey or maple syrup
- 1/2 teaspoon cinnamon
- Fresh fruit for topping

Possible Substitutes:
- Different plant-based milks
- Various sweeteners like agave nectar

Method of Preparation:
1. Rinse buckwheat groats under cold water.
2. In a saucepan, bring water to a boil and add buckwheat.
3. Reduce heat and simmer for 10-15 minutes until water is absorbed.
4. Stir in almond milk, honey, and cinnamon.
5. Cook for another 5 minutes until creamy.
6. Serve topped with fresh fruit.

Nutritional Value (per serving):

- Calories: 300
- Carbohydrates: 55g
- Protein: 8g
- Fat: 6g
- Fiber: 10g

Cost per Serving:
Approximately $2.00

"To eat well in England you should have breakfast three times a day."

– W. Somerset Maugham

Chapter 4: Lunch

1. QUINOA SALAD WITH CHICKPEAS AND VEGGIES

History:
Quinoa, known as the "mother grain" by the Incas, has been cultivated for over 5,000 years. This nutrient-rich grain has become a global superfood, valued for its high protein content and versatility.

Ingredients:
- 1 cup quinoa, cooked
- 1 can (15 oz) chickpeas, drained and rinsed
- 1 cup cherry tomatoes, halved
- 1 cucumber, diced
- 1/4 cup red onion, finely chopped
- 1/4 cup fresh parsley, chopped
- 1/4 cup olive oil
- 2 tablespoons lemon juice
- Salt and pepper to taste

Possible Substitutes:
- Different grains like farro or bulgur
- Black beans instead of chickpeas

Method of Preparation:
1. In a large bowl, combine cooked quinoa, chickpeas, cherry tomatoes, cucumber, red onion, and parsley.

2. In a small bowl, whisk together olive oil, lemon juice, salt, and pepper.
3. Pour the dressing over the salad and toss to combine.
4. Serve immediately or refrigerate for up to 2 days.

Nutritional Value (per serving):
- Calories: 320
- Carbohydrates: 45g
- Protein: 10g
- Fat: 12g
- Fiber: 8g

Cost per Serving:
Approximately $3.00

2. GRILLED CHICKEN SALAD

History:

Salads have been a dietary staple across many cultures. The grilled chicken salad offers a perfect blend of lean protein and fresh vegetables, making it a popular choice for a healthy lunch.

Ingredients:
- 2 chicken breasts
- 4 cups mixed greens (lettuce, spinach, arugula)
- 1 cup cherry tomatoes, halved
- 1 cucumber, sliced
- 1/4 cup red onion, thinly sliced
- 1/4 cup feta cheese, crumbled
- 1/4 cup olive oil
- 2 tablespoons balsamic vinegar
- Salt and pepper to taste

Possible Substitutes:
- Tofu or tempeh for a vegetarian option
- Goat cheese instead of feta

Method of Preparation:
1. Season chicken breasts with salt and pepper.
2. Grill the chicken over medium heat until fully cooked, about 6-8 minutes per side.
3. Let the chicken rest for a few minutes, then slice thinly.
4. In a large bowl, combine mixed greens, cherry tomatoes, cucumber, red onion, and feta cheese.

5. In a small bowl, whisk together olive oil and balsamic vinegar.
6. Toss the salad with the dressing and top with sliced chicken.
7. Serve immediately.

Nutritional Value (per serving):
- Calories: 350
- Carbohydrates: 10g
- Protein: 30g
- Fat: 20g
- Fiber: 3g

Cost per Serving:
Approximately $4.50

3. LENTIL SOUP

History:
Lentil soup has been enjoyed for millennia, with evidence of its consumption dating back to ancient Greece and Rome. This hearty, nutritious soup is a staple in many cultures due to its simplicity and health benefits.

Ingredients:
- 1 cup lentils, rinsed
- 1 onion, diced
- 2 carrots, diced
- 2 celery stalks, diced
- 3 cloves garlic, minced
- 1 can (14.5 oz) diced tomatoes
- 4 cups vegetable broth
- 1 teaspoon cumin
- 1 teaspoon paprika
- Salt and pepper to taste
- 2 tablespoons olive oil

Possible Substitutes:
- Different types of lentils
- Other root vegetables like sweet potatoes

Method of Preparation:
1. Heat olive oil in a large pot over medium heat.
2. Add onion, carrots, and celery, and sauté until softened.
3. Add garlic and cook for another minute.
4. Stir in lentils, diced tomatoes, vegetable broth, cumin, and paprika.

5. Bring to a boil, then reduce heat and simmer for 25-30 minutes, until lentils are tender.
6. Season with salt and pepper to taste.
7. Serve hot.

Nutritional Value (per serving):
- Calories: 250
- Carbohydrates: 35g
- Protein: 12g
- Fat: 7g
- Fiber: 12g

Cost per Serving:
Approximately $2.00

4. TURKEY AND AVOCADO WRAP

History:
Wraps are a modern twist on traditional sandwiches, providing a convenient and portable meal option. This turkey and avocado wrap combines lean protein with healthy fats for a balanced lunch.

Ingredients:
- 2 whole grain tortillas
- 4 slices deli turkey breast
- 1 avocado, sliced
- 1 cup baby spinach
- 1/4 cup hummus
- Salt and pepper to taste

Possible Substitutes:
- Chicken breast instead of turkey
- Different spreads like tzatziki or yogurt

Method of Preparation:
1. Lay out the tortillas and spread hummus evenly on each.
2. Layer turkey slices, avocado, and baby spinach on top.
3. Season with salt and pepper.
4. Roll up the tortillas tightly and slice in half.
5. Serve immediately or wrap in foil for later.

Nutritional Value (per serving):
- Calories: 350

- Carbohydrates: 30g
- Protein: 20g
- Fat: 18g
- Fiber: 8g

Cost per Serving:
Approximately $3.00

5. STUFFED BELL PEPPERS

History:
Stuffed bell peppers have origins in various cuisines, including Mediterranean and Latin American. They offer a versatile way to combine vegetables, grains, and proteins in a colourful, nutritious dish.

Ingredients:
- 4 bell peppers, tops cut off and seeds removed
- 1 cup cooked quinoa
- 1/2 cup black beans, drained and rinsed
- 1/2 cup corn kernels
- 1/2 cup diced tomatoes
- 1/4 cup chopped cilantro
- 1 teaspoon cumin
- 1 teaspoon chili powder
- Salt and pepper to taste
- 1/4 cup shredded cheese (optional)

Possible Substitutes:
- Brown rice instead of quinoa
- Different beans like pinto or kidney

Method of Preparation:
1. Preheat oven to 375°F (190°C).
2. In a large bowl, combine quinoa, black beans, corn, tomatoes, cilantro, cumin, chili powder, salt, and pepper.
3. Stuff each bell pepper with the quinoa mixture.

4. Place stuffed peppers in a baking dish and cover with foil.
5. Bake for 25-30 minutes, until peppers are tender.
6. Remove foil and sprinkle with cheese if desired, then bake for an additional 5 minutes.
7. Serve hot.

Nutritional Value (per serving):
- Calories: 300
- Carbohydrates: 45g
- Protein: 10g
- Fat: 8g
- Fiber: 10g

Cost per Serving:
Approximately $3.00

6. SPINACH AND FETA SALAD

History:
Spinach and feta salad is a classic combination in Greek cuisine, known for its fresh flavours and simple preparation. This salad is a great source of vitamins and minerals, especially iron and calcium.

Ingredients:
- 4 cups fresh spinach leaves
- 1/2 cup crumbled feta cheese
- 1/4 cup red onion, thinly sliced
- 1/4 cup kalamata olives, pitted and sliced
- 1/4 cup cherry tomatoes, halved
- 2 tablespoons olive oil
- 1 tablespoon red wine vinegar
- Salt and pepper to taste

Possible Substitutes:
- Arugula or mixed greens instead of spinach
- Goat cheese instead of feta

Method of Preparation:
1. In a large bowl, combine spinach, feta cheese, red onion, olives, and cherry tomatoes.
2. In a small bowl, whisk together olive oil, red wine vinegar, salt, and pepper.
3. Drizzle the dressing over the salad and toss to combine.
4. Serve immediately.

Nutritional Value (per serving):
- Calories: 200
- Carbohydrates: 8g
- Protein: 6g
- Fat: 18g
- Fiber: 4g

Cost per Serving:
Approximately $2.50

7. GREEK SALAD

History:
Greek salad, also known as horiatiki, is a staple of Greek cuisine. It typically features fresh vegetables, feta cheese, and olives, providing a refreshing and nutritious meal.

Ingredients:
- 4 cups chopped romaine lettuce
- 1 cucumber, sliced
- 1 cup cherry tomatoes, halved
- 1/2 red onion, thinly sliced
- 1/2 cup kalamata olives, pitted
- 1/2 cup crumbled feta cheese
- 1/4 cup olive oil
- 2 tablespoons red wine vinegar
- 1 teaspoon dried oregano
- Salt and pepper to taste

Possible Substitutes:
- Different greens like mixed lettuce
- Various olives for different flavours

Method of Preparation:
1. In a large bowl, combine romaine lettuce, cucumber, cherry tomatoes, red onion, olives, and feta cheese.
2. In a small bowl, whisk together olive oil, red wine vinegar, oregano, salt, and pepper.
3. Drizzle the dressing over the salad and toss to combine.
4. Serve immediately.

Nutritional Value (per serving):

- Calories: 250
- Carbohydrates: 10g
- Protein: 7g
- Fat: 22g
- Fiber: 4g

Cost per Serving:
Approximately $3.00

8. ROASTED VEGGIE AND HUMMUS WRAP

History:
Wraps are a versatile meal option that can incorporate various ingredients. Roasted veggies and hummus offer a flavourful and healthy combination, suitable for a quick and nutritious lunch.

Ingredients:
- 2 whole grain tortillas
- 1 cup mixed vegetables (bell peppers, zucchini, eggplant), sliced
- 1/4 cup hummus
- 1 tablespoon olive oil
- Salt and pepper to taste

Possible Substitutes:
- Different veggies like mushrooms or carrots
- Other spreads like avocado or yogurt

Method of Preparation:
1. Preheat oven to 400°F (200°C).
2. Toss sliced vegetables with olive oil, salt, and pepper.
3. Spread vegetables on a baking sheet and roast for 20-25 minutes, until tender.
4. Spread hummus on the tortillas.
5. Top with roasted vegetables.
6. Roll up the tortillas tightly and slice in half.
7. Serve immediately or wrap in foil for later.

Nutritional Value (per serving):

- Calories: 300
- Carbohydrates: 40g
- Protein: 8g
- Fat: 14g
- Fiber: 8g

Cost per Serving:
Approximately $2.50

9. TOFU STIR-FRY

History:
Stir-frying is a cooking technique originating in China, allowing for quick preparation of a variety of ingredients. Tofu stir-fry is a popular vegetarian option, providing a balanced and flavourful meal.

Ingredients:
- 1 block firm tofu, drained and cubed
- 1 cup broccoli florets
- 1 cup bell peppers, sliced
- 1 carrot, sliced
- 2 tablespoons soy sauce
- 1 tablespoon olive oil
- 2 cloves garlic, minced
- 1 teaspoon grated ginger
- Salt and pepper to taste

Possible Substitutes:
- Different vegetables like snow peas or bok choy
- Tamari instead of soy sauce for a gluten-free option

Method of Preparation:
1. Heat olive oil in a large skillet or wok over medium-high heat.
2. Add tofu cubes and cook until golden brown on all sides.
3. Remove tofu from the skillet and set aside.
4. Add garlic and ginger to the skillet, cooking for 1 minute.
5. Add broccoli, bell peppers, and carrot, and stir-fry for 5-7 minutes, until vegetables are tender.
6. Return tofu to the skillet and add soy sauce.

7. Stir to combine and cook for another 2 minutes.

8. Season with salt and pepper to taste.

9. Serve hot.

Nutritional Value (per serving):
- Calories: 250
- Carbohydrates: 15g
- Protein: 15g
- Fat: 14g
- Fiber: 5g

Cost per Serving:
Approximately $2.50

10. BLACK BEAN SOUP

History:
Black bean soup is a staple in Latin American cuisine, known for its hearty and nutritious qualities. It's a simple, flavourful dish that provides ample protein and fibre.

Ingredients:
- 2 cans (15 oz each) black beans, drained and rinsed
- 1 onion, diced
- 2 cloves garlic, minced
- 1 carrot, diced
- 1 celery stalk, diced
- 4 cups vegetable broth
- 1 teaspoon cumin
- 1 teaspoon paprika
- 1 tablespoon olive oil
- Salt and pepper to taste

Possible Substitutes:
- Different beans like kidney or pinto
- Chicken broth instead of vegetable broth

Method of Preparation:
1. Heat olive oil in a large pot over medium heat.
2. Add onion, carrot, and celery, and sauté until softened.
3. Add garlic and cook for another minute.
4. Stir in black beans, vegetable broth, cumin, and paprika.
5. Bring to a boil, then reduce heat and simmer for 20 minutes.
6. Use an immersion blender to partially blend the soup, leaving some chunks for texture.

7. Season with salt and pepper to taste.
8. Serve hot.

Nutritional Value (per serving):
- Calories: 300
- Carbohydrates: 45g
- Protein: 15g
- Fat: 8g
- Fiber: 15g

Cost per Serving:
Approximately $2.00

Chapter 5: Dinner

1. GRILLED SALMON WITH ASPARAGUS

History:
Salmon has been a vital food source for many coastal cultures, prized for its rich flavour and high omega-3 content. Paired with asparagus, a spring vegetable known for its delicate taste and nutritional benefits, this dish is both delicious and healthful.

Ingredients:
- 2 salmon fillets
- 1 bunch asparagus, trimmed
- 2 tablespoons olive oil
- 1 lemon, sliced
- Salt and pepper to taste

Possible Substitutes:
- Other fish like trout or cod
- Green beans instead of asparagus

Method of Preparation:
1. Preheat the grill to medium-high heat.
2. Drizzle salmon and asparagus with olive oil and season with salt and pepper.
3. Place salmon and asparagus on the grill.
4. Grill salmon for 4-5 minutes per side until fully cooked.
5. Grill asparagus for 5-7 minutes until tender.
6. Serve salmon and asparagus with lemon slices.

Nutritional Value (per serving):

- Calories: 400
- Carbohydrates: 8g
- Protein: 35g
- Fat: 25g
- Fiber: 4g

Cost per Serving:
Approximately $6.00

2. VEGETABLE STIR-FRY WITH TOFU

History:
Stir-frying is a quick cooking technique that originated in China. This method allows vegetables and proteins to retain their nutrients and vibrant colors, making it a healthy and visually appealing dish.

Ingredients:
- 1 block firm tofu, cubed
- 1 cup broccoli florets
- 1 red bell pepper, sliced
- 1 carrot, sliced
- 2 tablespoons soy sauce
- 1 tablespoon olive oil
- 2 cloves garlic, minced
- 1 teaspoon grated ginger
- Salt and pepper to taste

Possible Substitutes:
- Chicken or shrimp instead of tofu
- Any other vegetables like snow peas or baby corn

Method of Preparation:
1. Heat olive oil in a large skillet over medium-high heat.
2. Add tofu cubes and cook until golden brown on all sides.
3. Remove tofu from skillet and set aside.
4. Add garlic and ginger to the skillet and cook for 1 minute.
5. Add broccoli, bell pepper, and carrot, stir-frying for 5-7

minutes until tender.

6. Return tofu to the skillet and add soy sauce.

7. Stir to combine and cook for another 2 minutes.

8. Season with salt and pepper to taste and serve hot.

Nutritional Value (per serving):
- Calories: 250
- Carbohydrates: 15g
- Protein: 15g
- Fat: 14g
- Fiber: 5g

Cost per Serving:
Approximately $3.00

3. CHICKEN AND BROCCOLI BAKE

History:
Casseroles and bakes have been popular in American cuisine for their convenience and ability to feed a family. This chicken and broccoli bake is a healthier take, providing lean protein and vegetables in a comforting dish.

Ingredients:
- 2 chicken breasts, diced
- 2 cups broccoli florets
- 1 cup shredded cheese (cheddar or mozzarella)
- 1/2 cup Greek yogurt
- 1/2 cup chicken broth
- 1 tablespoon olive oil
- Salt and pepper to taste

Possible Substitutes:
- Cauliflower instead of broccoli
- Plant-based cheese for a dairy-free option

Method of Preparation:
1. Preheat oven to 375°F (190°C).
2. Heat olive oil in a skillet over medium heat.
3. Add chicken and cook until browned.
4. In a large bowl, mix chicken, broccoli, Greek yogurt, chicken broth, salt, and pepper.
5. Transfer to a baking dish and top with shredded cheese.
6. Bake for 25-30 minutes until cheese is melted and bubbly.

7. Serve hot.

Nutritional Value (per serving):
- Calories: 350
- Carbohydrates: 10g
- Protein: 35g
- Fat: 18g
- Fiber: 4g

Cost per Serving:
Approximately $4.00

4. BEEF AND VEGETABLE STEW

History:
Stews have been a part of culinary traditions worldwide for centuries, known for their hearty and warming qualities. This beef and vegetable stew is a comforting meal that provides a balanced mix of protein and vegetables.

Ingredients:
- 1 lb beef stew meat, cubed
- 2 carrots, diced
- 2 potatoes, diced
- 1 onion, diced
- 2 cloves garlic, minced
- 4 cups beef broth
- 1 tablespoon olive oil
- 1 teaspoon thyme
- 1 teaspoon rosemary
- Salt and pepper to taste

Possible Substitutes:
- Lamb or chicken instead of beef
- Sweet potatoes instead of regular potatoes

Method of Preparation:
1. Heat olive oil in a large pot over medium heat.
2. Add beef and brown on all sides.
3. Remove beef from pot and set aside.
4. Add onion, carrots, and potatoes to the pot, cooking until

softened.

5. Add garlic and cook for another minute.

6. Return beef to the pot and add beef broth, thyme, rosemary, salt, and pepper.

7. Bring to a boil, then reduce heat and simmer for 1-2 hours until beef is tender.

8. Serve hot.

Nutritional Value (per serving):
- Calories: 400
- Carbohydrates: 25g
- Protein: 30g
- Fat: 18g
- Fiber: 6g

Cost per Serving:
Approximately $5.00

5. CAULIFLOWER RICE STIR-FRY

History:
Cauliflower rice has gained popularity as a low-carb alternative to traditional rice. This stir-fry combines the versatility of cauliflower with the vibrant flavours of Asian cuisine.

Ingredients:
- 1 head cauliflower, grated into rice-sized pieces
- 1 cup mixed vegetables (carrots, peas, bell peppers)
- 2 eggs, beaten
- 2 tablespoons soy sauce
- 1 tablespoon olive oil
- 2 cloves garlic, minced
- 1 teaspoon grated ginger
- Salt and pepper to taste

Possible Substitutes:
- Broccoli rice instead of cauliflower rice
- Tamari for a gluten-free option

Method of Preparation:
1. Heat olive oil in a large skillet over medium-high heat.
2. Add garlic and ginger, cooking for 1 minute.
3. Add mixed vegetables and stir-fry for 5-7 minutes until tender.
4. Push vegetables to one side of the skillet and pour beaten eggs into the other side, scrambling them.
5. Add grated cauliflower and soy sauce, stirring to combine.

6. Cook for another 3-5 minutes until cauliflower is tender.
7. Season with salt and pepper to taste and serve hot.

Nutritional Value (per serving):
- Calories: 200
- Carbohydrates: 15g
- Protein: 10g
- Fat: 12g
- Fiber: 5g

Cost per Serving:
Approximately $2.00

6. BAKED COD WITH TOMATOES AND OLIVES

History:
Cod has been a staple in many coastal diets due to its mild flavour and flaky texture. This Mediterranean-inspired dish combines cod with tomatoes and olives for a light yet flavourful meal.

Ingredients:
- 2 cod fillets
- 1 cup cherry tomatoes, halved
- 1/2 cup kalamata olives, pitted and sliced
- 1 lemon, sliced
- 2 tablespoons olive oil
- 1 teaspoon dried oregano
- Salt and pepper to taste

Possible Substitutes:
- Other white fish like haddock or halibut
- Capers instead of olives

Method of Preparation:
1. Preheat oven to 375°F (190°C).
2. Place cod fillets in a baking dish and top with cherry tomatoes, olives, and lemon slices.
3. Drizzle with olive oil and season with oregano, salt, and

pepper.
4. Bake for 20-25 minutes until cod is cooked through and flakes easily with a fork.
5. Serve hot.

Nutritional Value (per serving):
- Calories: 300
- Carbohydrates: 10g
- Protein: 30g
- Fat: 15g
- Fiber: 3g

Cost per Serving:
Approximately $4.00

7. ZUCCHINI NOODLES WITH PESTO

History:
Zucchini noodles, or zoodles, have become a popular low-carb alternative to pasta. Paired with pesto, this dish offers a fresh and healthy take on traditional Italian flavours.

Ingredients:
- 2 large zucchinis, spiralized
- 1/2 cup basil pesto
- 1/4 cup cherry tomatoes, halved
- 2 tablespoons olive oil
- Salt and pepper to taste

Possible Substitutes:
- Spaghetti squash instead of zucchini
- Different types of pesto, like spinach or arugula

Method of Preparation:
1. Heat olive oil in a large skillet over medium heat.
2. Add zucchini noodles and sauté for 3-5 minutes until tender.
3. Add pesto and cherry tomatoes, tossing to combine.
4. Cook for another 2 minutes until heated through.
5. Season with salt and

pepper to taste and serve hot.

Nutritional Value (per serving):
- Calories: 250
- Carbohydrates: 10g
- Protein: 6g
- Fat: 22g
- Fiber: 4g

Cost per Serving:
Approximately $3.00

8. EGGPLANT PARMESAN

History:
Eggplant Parmesan, or Parmigiana di Melanzane, is a classic Italian dish. This version is baked instead of fried, offering a lighter but equally delicious alternative.

Ingredients:
- 1 large eggplant, sliced into rounds
- 2 cups marinara sauce
- 1 cup shredded mozzarella cheese
- 1/2 cup grated Parmesan cheese
- 1/2 cup whole wheat breadcrumbs
- 2 eggs, beaten
- 1 tablespoon olive oil
- Salt and pepper to taste

Possible Substitutes:
- Zucchini instead of eggplant
- Vegan cheese for a dairy-free option

Method of Preparation:
1. Preheat oven to 375°F (190°C).
2. Dip eggplant slices in beaten eggs, then coat with breadcrumbs.
3. Place eggplant slices on a baking sheet and drizzle with olive oil.
4. Bake for 20 minutes, flipping halfway through, until golden brown.

5. In a baking dish, spread a layer of marinara sauce and top with eggplant slices.

6. Sprinkle with mozzarella and Parmesan cheese.

7. Repeat layers until all ingredients are used, ending with cheese on top.

8. Bake for 25-30 minutes until cheese is melted and bubbly.

9. Serve hot.

Nutritional Value (per serving):
- Calories: 350
- Carbohydrates: 30g
- Protein: 15g
- Fat: 20g
- Fiber: 7g

Cost per Serving:
Approximately $4.00

9. TURKEY MEATBALLS WITH ZUCCHINI NOODLES

History:
Turkey meatballs offer a leaner alternative to traditional beef meatballs. Paired with zucchini noodles, this dish provides a nutritious and low-carb option for pasta lovers.

Ingredients:
- 1 lb ground turkey
- 1/4 cup grated Parmesan cheese
- 1/4 cup whole wheat breadcrumbs
- 1 egg
- 2 cloves garlic, minced
- 1 teaspoon dried oregano
- 2 large zucchinis, spiralized
- 2 cups marinara sauce
- 2 tablespoons olive oil
- Salt and pepper to taste

Possible Substitutes:
- Ground chicken instead of turkey
- Spaghetti squash instead of zucchini

Method of Preparation:
1. In a bowl, combine ground turkey, Parmesan cheese, breadcrumbs, egg, garlic, oregano, salt, and pepper.

2. Form mixture into meatballs.
3. Heat 1 tablespoon olive oil in a large skillet over medium heat.
4. Cook meatballs until browned on all sides and cooked through.
5. In another skillet, heat 1 tablespoon olive oil and sauté zucchini noodles for 3-5 minutes until tender.
6. Add marinara sauce to the meatballs and simmer for 5 minutes.
7. Serve meatballs and sauce over zucchini noodles.

Nutritional Value (per serving):
- Calories: 350
- Carbohydrates: 15g
- Protein: 30g
- Fat: 18g
- Fiber: 5g

Cost per Serving:
Approximately $3.50

10. SHRIMP AND VEGGIE SKEWERS

History:
Grilling skewers is a cooking technique found in many cultures, offering a versatile way to prepare meat and vegetables. Shrimp skewers are popular for their quick cooking time and delicious flavour.

Ingredients:
- 1 lb large shrimp, peeled and deveined
- 1 red bell pepper, cut into chunks
- 1 zucchini, sliced
- 1 red onion, cut into chunks
- 2 tablespoons olive oil
- 2 cloves garlic, minced
- 1 lemon, juiced
- Salt and pepper to taste

Possible Substitutes:
- Chicken or tofu instead of shrimp
- Any other vegetables like mushrooms or cherry tomatoes

Method of Preparation:
1. Preheat the grill to medium-high heat.
2. In a bowl, combine olive oil, garlic, lemon juice, salt, and pepper.
3. Thread shrimp, bell pepper, zucchini, and red onion onto skewers.
4. Brush with olive oil mixture.

5. Grill skewers for 2-3 minutes per side until shrimp is cooked through and vegetables are tender.
6. Serve hot.

Nutritional Value (per serving):
- Calories: 250
- Carbohydrates: 10g
- Protein: 25g
- Fat: 12g
- Fiber: 3g

Cost per Serving:
Approximately $4.00

Chapter 6: Snacks

1. HUMMUS WITH VEGGIE STICKS

History:
Hummus, a staple of Middle Eastern cuisine, dates back to ancient Egypt. This nutritious dip is made from chickpeas and tahini and has gained worldwide popularity for its versatility and health benefits.

Ingredients:
- 1 can (15 oz) chickpeas, drained and rinsed
- 1/4 cup tahini
- 2 tablespoons olive oil
- 1 lemon, juiced
- 2 cloves garlic, minced
- Salt and pepper to taste
- Assorted veggie sticks (carrots, celery, bell peppers, cucumber)

Possible Substitutes:
- White beans or black beans instead of chickpeas
- Sunflower seed butter instead of tahini

Method of Preparation:
1. In a food processor, combine chickpeas, tahini, olive oil, lemon juice, garlic, salt, and pepper.
2. Blend until smooth, adding water if needed to reach desired consistency.
3. Serve hummus with assorted veggie sticks.

Nutritional Value (per serving):

- Calories: 200
- Carbohydrates: 20g
- Protein: 6g
- Fat: 12g
- Fiber: 6g

Cost per Serving:
Approximately $2.00

2. BAKED SWEET POTATO FRIES

History:
Sweet potatoes are native to Central and South America and have been cultivated for thousands of years. Baked sweet potato fries offer a healthier alternative to traditional fries, providing fibre and vitamins.

Ingredients:
- 2 large, sweet potatoes, peeled and cut into fries
- 2 tablespoons olive oil
- 1 teaspoon paprika
- 1/2 teaspoon garlic powder
- Salt and pepper to taste

Possible Substitutes:
- Regular potatoes or carrots for variety

Method of Preparation:
1. Preheat oven to 425°F (220°C).
2. In a large bowl, toss sweet potato fries with olive oil, paprika, garlic powder, salt, and pepper.
3. Spread fries in a single layer on a baking sheet.
4. Bake for 25-30 minutes, turning halfway, until crispy.
5. Serve hot.

Nutritional Value (per serving):
- Calories: 180
- Carbohydrates: 30g

- Protein: 2g
- Fat: 6g
- Fiber: 5g

Cost per Serving:
Approximately $1.50

3. GREEK YOGURT WITH HONEY AND NUTS

History:
Greek yogurt, known for its creamy texture and high protein content, has been a staple in Mediterranean diets for centuries. This snack combines the yogurt with honey and nuts for added flavour and nutrition.

Ingredients:
- 1 cup Greek yogurt
- 1 tablespoon honey
- 1/4 cup mixed nuts (almonds, walnuts, pistachios)

Possible Substitutes:
- Plant-based yogurt for a dairy-free option
- Seeds instead of nuts

Method of Preparation:
1. Scoop Greek yogurt into a bowl.
2. Drizzle with honey.
3. Top with mixed nuts.
4. Serve immediately.

Nutritional Value (per serving):
- Calories: 250
- Carbohydrates: 20g
- Protein: 15g

- Fat: 12g
- Fiber: 2g

Cost per Serving:
Approximately $2.50

4. MIXED NUTS AND SEEDS

History:
Nuts and seeds have been consumed by humans since prehistoric times. They are rich in healthy fats, protein, and various essential nutrients, making them a perfect snack for sustained energy.

Ingredients:
- 1/2 cup almonds
- 1/2 cup walnuts
- 1/2 cup pumpkin seeds
- 1/2 cup sunflower seeds
- 1/4 cup chia seeds

Possible Substitutes:
- Any combination of your favourite nuts and seeds

Method of Preparation:
1. Mix all nuts and seeds in a large bowl.
2. Store in an airtight container.
3. Serve as a snack.

Nutritional Value (per serving):
- Calories: 200
- Carbohydrates: 10g
- Protein: 6g
- Fat: 18g
- Fiber: 4g

Cost per Serving:
Approximately $2.00

5. FRUIT SALAD

History:
Fruit salads have been enjoyed in various forms around the world for centuries. They provide a refreshing and nutritious way to consume a variety of fruits.

Ingredients:
- 1 cup strawberries, sliced
- 1 cup blueberries
- 1 cup pineapple chunks
- 1 apple, diced
- 1 banana, sliced
- 1 tablespoon lemon juice

Possible Substitutes:
- Any seasonal fruits

Method of Preparation:
1. In a large bowl, combine all the fruits.
2. Drizzle with lemon juice and toss gently.
3. Serve immediately or refrigerate until ready to serve.

Nutritional Value (per serving):
- Calories: 150
- Carbohydrates: 35g
- Protein: 2g
- Fat: 1g
- Fiber: 7g

Cost per Serving:
Approximately $2.50

6. KALE CHIPS

History:
Kale has been cultivated for over 2,000 years and has gained popularity in recent years as a superfood. Kale chips provide a crispy and healthy alternative to potato chips.

Ingredients:
- 1 bunch kale, stems removed and leaves torn into pieces
- 2 tablespoons olive oil
- Salt and pepper to taste

Possible Substitutes:
- Spinach or Swiss chard for variety

Method of Preparation:
1. Preheat oven to 300°F (150°C).
2. In a large bowl, toss kale with olive oil, salt, and pepper.
3. Spread kale in a single layer on a baking sheet.
4. Bake for 20-25 minutes until crispy, turning halfway through.
5. Serve immediately.

Nutritional Value (per serving):
- Calories: 100
- Carbohydrates: 7g
- Protein: 3g
- Fat: 7g
- Fiber: 3g

Cost per Serving:
Approximately $1.50

7. APPLE SLICES WITH ALMOND BUTTER

History:
Apples have been a staple fruit for thousands of years, and almond butter is a nutritious spread made from ground almonds. This combination provides a balanced snack with fibre and healthy fats.

Ingredients:
- 1 apple, sliced
- 2 tablespoons almond butter

Possible Substitutes:
- Peanut butter or sunflower seed butter

Method of Preparation:
1. Core and slice the apple.
2. Serve apple slices with almond butter for dipping.

Nutritional Value (per serving):
- Calories: 200
- Carbohydrates: 25g
- Protein: 4g
- Fat: 10g
- Fiber: 5g

Cost per Serving:
Approximately $1.50

8. EDAMAME

History:
Edamame, young soybeans, have been a popular snack in East Asian cuisine for centuries. They are rich in protein and fibre, making them a healthy snack option.

Ingredients:
- 1 cup edamame (in the pod)
- 1 teaspoon sea salt

Possible Substitutes:
- Green peas for a similar snack

Method of Preparation:
1. Boil edamame in salted water for 5 minutes.
2. Drain and sprinkle with sea salt.
3. Serve hot or cold.

Nutritional Value (per serving):
- Calories: 120
- Carbohydrates: 10g
- Protein: 12g
- Fat: 5g
- Fiber: 5g

Cost per Serving:
Approximately $2.00

9. COTTAGE CHEESE WITH CUCUMBERS AND TOMATOES

History:
Cottage cheese has been a part of various culinary traditions for centuries, valued for its high protein content. Combining it with fresh vegetables makes for a refreshing and nutritious snack.

Ingredients:
- 1 cup cottage cheese
- 1/2 cup cucumber, diced
- 1/2 cup cherry tomatoes, halved
- Salt and pepper to taste

Possible Substitutes:
- Greek yogurt instead of cottage cheese

Method of Preparation:
1. In a bowl, combine cottage cheese, cucumber, and cherry tomatoes.
2. Season with salt and pepper.
3. Serve immediately.

Nutritional Value (per serving):
- Calories: 200
- Carbohydrates: 10g
- Protein: 20g
- Fat: 8g

- Fiber: 2g

Cost per Serving:
Approximately $2.00

10. GUACAMOLE WITH BELL PEPPER SLICES

History:
Guacamole, originating from Mexico, is a popular dip made from avocados. It is rich in healthy fats and vitamins. Paired with bell pepper slices, it makes for a colourful and nutritious snack.

Ingredients:
- 2 ripe avocados, mashed
- 1 lime, juiced
- 1/4 cup red onion, finely chopped
- 1/4 cup cilantro, chopped
- Salt and pepper to taste
- Assorted bell pepper slices

Possible Substitutes:
- Greek yogurt mixed with avocado for a creamier dip

Method of Preparation:
1. In a bowl, combine mashed avocados, lime juice, red onion, cilantro, salt, and pepper.
2. Mix well until smooth.
3. Serve guacamole with bell pepper slices.

Nutritional Value (per serving):
- Calories: 250
- Carbohydrates: 20g

- Protein: 3g
- Fat: 20g
- Fiber: 10g

Cost per Serving:
Approximately $2.50

Chapter 7: Drinks

1. GREEN SMOOTHIE

History:
Green smoothies have become popular in recent years as part of health and wellness trends. They provide a convenient way to consume leafy greens and other nutritious ingredients in a tasty and refreshing form.

Ingredients:
- 1 cup spinach leaves
- 1 banana
- 1/2 cup frozen mango
- 1/2 cup almond milk
- 1 tablespoon chia seeds

Possible Substitutes:
- Kale instead of spinach
- Different fruits like pineapple or berries

Method of Preparation:
1. Combine spinach, banana, frozen mango, and almond milk in a blender.
2. Blend until smooth.
3. Pour into a glass and sprinkle with chia seeds.
4. Serve immediately.

Nutritional Value (per serving):
- Calories: 200
- Carbohydrates: 40g
- Protein: 4g
- Fat: 5g
- Fiber: 8g

**Cost per Serving:
Approximately $2.50**

2. HERBAL ICED TEA

History:
Herbal teas have been used for their medicinal properties for centuries. Iced herbal tea provides a refreshing way to enjoy these benefits, especially in warmer weather.

Ingredients:
- 4 cups water
- 4 herbal tea bags (such as chamomile, peppermint, or hibiscus)
- 1 lemon, sliced
- 1 tablespoon honey or stevia (optional)
- Ice cubes

Possible Substitutes:
- Any preferred herbal tea variety

Method of Preparation:
1. Boil water and steep tea bags for 5-7 minutes.
2. Remove tea bags and let the tea cool to room temperature.
3. Add honey or stevia if desired.
4. Pour tea over ice in a pitcher.
5. Add lemon slices and serve chilled.

Nutritional Value (per serving):
- Calories: 10 (without sweetener)
- Carbohydrates: 3g
- Protein: 0g
- Fat: 0g
- Fiber: 0g

Cost per Serving:

Approximately $1.00

3. COCONUT WATER

History:
Coconut water has been a staple in tropical regions for centuries, valued for its hydrating properties and natural electrolytes. It has become popular worldwide as a refreshing and healthy beverage.

Ingredients:
- 1 fresh coconut or 1 cup bottled coconut water

Possible Substitutes:
- None for true coconut water

Method of Preparation:
1. If using a fresh coconut, pierce the top and pour the water into a glass.
2. Serve chilled.

Nutritional Value (per serving):
- Calories: 45
- Carbohydrates: 9g
- Protein: 1g
- Fat: 0g
- Fiber: 1g

Cost per Serving:
Approximately $2.00

4. ALMOND MILK LATTE

History:
Almond milk has been used as a dairy alternative for centuries. Combined with coffee, it makes a creamy and delicious latte suitable for those avoiding dairy.

Ingredients:
- 1 cup almond milk
- 1 shot espresso or 1/2 cup strong brewed coffee
- 1 teaspoon vanilla extract
- 1 teaspoon honey or stevia (optional)

Possible Substitutes:
- Other plant-based milks like soy or oat milk

Method of Preparation:
1. Heat almond milk in a saucepan until warm (do not boil).
2. Brew espresso or strong coffee.
3. Froth the warm almond milk using a milk frothier or whisk.
4. Pour the coffee into a mug and add the frothed almond milk.
5. Stir in vanilla extract and honey or stevia if desired.
6. Serve immediately.

Nutritional Value (per serving):
- Calories: 60
- Carbohydrates: 5g
- Protein: 2g
- Fat: 4g

- Fiber: 1g

Cost per Serving:
Approximately $1.50

5. BERRY INFUSED WATER

History:
Infusing water with fruits has been a traditional practice to enhance the flavour and encourage hydration. Berry-infused water is both refreshing and packed with vitamins.

Ingredients:
- 1 cup mixed berries (strawberries, blueberries, raspberries)
- 4 cups water
- Ice cubes
- Fresh mint leaves (optional)

Possible Substitutes:
- Any preferred fruits for infusion

Method of Preparation:
1. Place berries in a pitcher and lightly mash with a spoon to release juices.
2. Fill the pitcher with water and add ice cubes.
3. Add mint leaves if desired.
4. Let the water infuse in the refrigerator for at least 1 hour.
5. Serve chilled.

Nutritional Value (per serving):
- Calories: 10
- Carbohydrates: 2g
- Protein: 0g
- Fat: 0g

- Fiber: 0g

Cost per Serving:
Approximately $1.00

6. GINGER LEMON TEA

History:
Ginger and lemon have been used in traditional medicine for their soothing and detoxifying properties. This tea combines the two for a refreshing and healthful beverage.

Ingredients:
- 4 cups water
- 1-inch piece of fresh ginger, sliced
- 1 lemon, juiced
- 1 tablespoon honey or stevia (optional)

Possible Substitutes:
- Ground ginger instead of fresh ginger

Method of Preparation:
1. Boil water and add sliced ginger.
2. Simmer for 10 minutes.
3. Remove from heat and add lemon juice.
4. Stir in honey or stevia if desired.
5. Serve hot or chilled over ice.

Nutritional Value (per serving):
- Calories: 20
- Carbohydrates: 5g
- Protein: 0g
- Fat: 0g
- Fiber: 0g

Cost per Serving:
Approximately $1.50

7. GREEN TEA WITH MINT

History:
Green tea has been consumed in Asia for thousands of years for its antioxidant properties. Adding mint enhances its refreshing qualities and provides additional health benefits.

Ingredients:
- 4 cups water
- 4 green tea bags
- 1/4 cup fresh mint leaves
- 1 tablespoon honey or stevia (optional)
- Ice cubes

Possible Substitutes:
- Any preferred tea variety

Method of Preparation:
1. Boil water and steep green tea bags and mint leaves for 3-5 minutes.
2. Remove tea bags and mint leaves, and let the tea cool to room temperature.
3. Add honey or stevia if desired.
4. Pour tea over ice in a pitcher.
5. Serve chilled.

Nutritional Value (per serving):
- Calories: 10 (without sweetener)
- Carbohydrates: 3g

- Protein: 0g
- Fat: 0g
- Fiber: 0g

Cost per Serving:
Approximately $1.50

8. CUCUMBER AND MINT WATER

History:
Cucumber and mint water is a classic spa beverage known for its hydrating and cooling effects. It's simple to prepare and helps encourage increased water intake.

Ingredients:
- 1 cucumber, thinly sliced
- 1/4 cup fresh mint leaves
- 4 cups water
- Ice cubes

Possible Substitutes:
- Lemon slices for added flavour

Method of Preparation:
1. Place cucumber slices and mint leaves in a pitcher.
2. Fill the pitcher with water and add ice cubes.
3. Let the water infuse in the refrigerator for at least 1 hour.
4. Serve chilled.

Nutritional Value (per serving):
- Calories: 5
- Carbohydrates: 1g
- Protein: 0g
- Fat: 0g
- Fiber: 0g

Cost per Serving:

Approximately $1.00

9. TOMATO JUICE

History:
Tomato juice has been a popular beverage since the early 20th century, valued for its rich flavour and high vitamin content. It is often consumed as a refreshing drink or used as a base for cocktails.

Ingredients:
- 4 large tomatoes, chopped
- 1 celery stalk, chopped
- 1/4 cup fresh parsley
- 1 tablespoon lemon juice
- Salt and pepper to taste

Possible Substitutes:
- Store-bought low-sodium tomato juice

Method of Preparation:
1. In a blender, combine tomatoes, celery, parsley, and lemon juice.
2. Blend until smooth.
3. Strain the juice through a fine mesh sieve to remove pulp.
4. Season with salt and pepper to taste.
5. Serve chilled.

Nutritional Value (per serving):
- Calories: 50
- Carbohydrates: 10g
- Protein: 2g
- Fat: 0g
- Fiber: 2g

Cost per Serving:
Approximately $2.00

10. CHIA SEED LEMONADE

History:
Chia seeds, once a staple of the Aztec diet, are known for their high omega-3 and fibre content. Adding them to lemonade creates a unique and nutritious beverage.

Ingredients:
- 4 cups water
- 1/4 cup lemon juice
- 2 tablespoons chia

seeds
- 1 tablespoon honey or stevia (optional)
- Ice cubes

Possible Substitutes:
- Lime juice for a different flavour

Method of Preparation:
1. In a pitcher, combine water, lemon juice, chia seeds, and honey or stevia if desired.
2. Stir well and let sit for 10 minutes, stirring occasionally to prevent chia seeds from clumping.
3. Add ice cubes and serve chilled.

Nutritional Value (per serving):
- Calories: 30
- Carbohydrates: 5g
- Protein: 1g

- Fat: 1g
- Fiber: 4g

Cost per Serving:
Approximately $2.00

Chapter 8: Special Occasions

1. STUFFED TURKEY BREAST

History:
Stuffed turkey breast is a modern twist on the traditional holiday turkey, offering a more manageable and quicker cooking alternative while still delivering the flavours and festivity of a whole roasted turkey.

Ingredients:
- 1 large turkey breast, butterflied
- 1 cup spinach, chopped
- 1/2 cup sun-dried tomatoes, chopped
- 1/2 cup feta cheese, crumbled
- 2 cloves garlic, minced
- 2 tablespoons olive oil
- Salt and pepper to taste

Possible Substitutes:
- Chicken breast instead of turkey
- Goat cheese instead of feta

Method of Preparation:
1. Preheat oven to 375°F (190°C).
2. In a skillet, heat olive oil and sauté garlic until fragrant.
3. Add spinach and sun-dried tomatoes, cooking until spinach is wilted.
4. Remove from heat and stir in feta cheese.
5. Lay the turkey breast flat and spread the spinach mixture over it.

6. Roll up the turkey breast and secure with kitchen twine.
7. Place the stuffed turkey breast in a baking dish and roast for 45-55 minutes until fully cooked.
8. Let rest for 10 minutes before slicing and serving.

Nutritional Value (per serving):
- Calories: 350
- Carbohydrates: 5g
- Protein: 50g
- Fat: 15g
- Fiber: 2g

Cost per Serving:
Approximately $5.00

2. VEGETABLE LASAGNA

History:
Lasagna is an Italian dish that has been enjoyed for centuries. This vegetable version provides a lighter and healthier alternative, packed with layers of vegetables, cheese, and whole grain pasta.

Ingredients:
- 9 whole wheat lasagna noodles
- 2 cups ricotta cheese
- 2 cups mozzarella cheese, shredded
- 1/2 cup Parmesan cheese, grated
- 1 zucchini, sliced
- 1 yellow squash, sliced
- 1 red bell pepper, sliced
- 2 cups spinach, chopped
- 4 cups marinara sauce
- 2 tablespoons olive oil
- Salt and pepper to taste

Possible Substitutes:
- Gluten-free lasagna noodles
- Different vegetables like eggplant or mushrooms

Method of Preparation:
1. Preheat oven to 375°F (190°C).
2. Cook lasagna noodles according to package instructions.
3. In a skillet, heat olive oil and sauté zucchini, squash, and bell

pepper until tender.

4. In a baking dish, spread a layer of marinara sauce, followed by a layer of noodles.

5. Spread ricotta cheese over the noodles, then top with sautéed vegetables and spinach.

6. Sprinkle with mozzarella and Parmesan cheese.

7. Repeat layers, ending with a layer of marinara sauce and cheese.

8. Cover with foil and bake for 30 minutes.

9. Remove foil and bake for an additional 15 minutes until cheese is bubbly and golden.

10. Let rest for 10 minutes before serving.

Nutritional Value (per serving):
- Calories: 400
- Carbohydrates: 45g
- Protein: 20g
- Fat: 18g
- Fiber: 8g

Cost per Serving:
Approximately $4.00

3. PUMPKIN PIE

History:
Pumpkin pie is a classic American dessert, especially popular during Thanksgiving. Made from spiced pumpkin filling in a pastry crust, it has been enjoyed for centuries as a comforting holiday treat.

Ingredients:
- 1 9-inch whole wheat pie crust
- 2 cups pumpkin puree
- 1 cup almond milk
- 1/2 cup maple syrup
- 2 eggs
- 1 teaspoon cinnamon
- 1/2 teaspoon ginger
- 1/2 teaspoon nutmeg
- 1/4 teaspoon cloves
- 1/4 teaspoon salt

Possible Substitutes:
- Coconut milk instead of almond milk
- Sweet potato puree instead of pumpkin

Method of Preparation:
1. Preheat oven to 350°F (175°C).
2. In a large bowl, whisk together pumpkin puree, almond milk, maple syrup, eggs, cinnamon, ginger, nutmeg, cloves, and salt until smooth.
3. Pour the filling into the pie crust.
4. Bake for 50-60 minutes until the filling is set.

5. Let cool completely before serving.

Nutritional Value (per serving):
- Calories: 250
- Carbohydrates: 35g
- Protein: 5g
- Fat: 10g
- Fiber: 5g

Cost per Serving:
Approximately $2.50

4. ROASTED VEGGIE PLATTER

History:
Roasting vegetables is a simple and ancient cooking method that enhances their natural flavours. A roasted veggie platter is a versatile dish perfect for any special occasion, showcasing a variety of colourful and nutritious vegetables.

Ingredients:
- 1 red bell pepper, sliced
- 1 yellow bell pepper, sliced
- 1 zucchini, sliced
- 1 yellow squash, sliced
- 1 red onion, sliced
- 1 cup cherry tomatoes
- 2 tablespoons olive oil
- 1 teaspoon dried oregano
- 1 teaspoon dried thyme
- Salt and pepper to taste

Possible Substitutes:
- Any seasonal vegetables

Method of Preparation:
1. Preheat oven to 400°F (200°C).
2. In a large bowl, toss all the vegetables with olive oil, oregano, thyme, salt, and pepper.
3. Spread the vegetables in a single layer on a baking sheet.
4. Roast for 20-25 minutes until tender and slightly charred.

5. Serve hot or at room temperature.

Nutritional Value (per serving):
- Calories: 150
- Carbohydrates: 15g
- Protein: 3g
- Fat: 9g
- Fiber: 5g

Cost per Serving:
Approximately $2.00

5. BAKED STUFFED APPLES

History:
Baked stuffed apples are a traditional dessert in many cultures, often enjoyed during the fall and winter months. This dish combines the natural sweetness of apples with a spiced filling, making it a perfect treat for special occasions.

Ingredients:
- 4 large apples, cored
- 1/4 cup rolled oats
- 1/4 cup chopped walnuts
- 2 tablespoons raisins
- 2 tablespoons honey
- 1 teaspoon cinnamon
- 1/2 teaspoon nutmeg
- 1 tablespoon butter, melted

Possible Substitutes:
- Almonds or pecans instead of walnuts
- Dried cranberries instead of raisins

Method of Preparation:
1. Preheat oven to 350°F (175°C).
2. In a bowl, combine oats, walnuts, raisins, honey, cinnamon, nutmeg, and melted butter.
3. Stuff the mixture into the cored apples.
4. Place apples in a baking dish and add a little water to the bottom of the dish.

5. Bake for 25-30 minutes until apples are tender.
6. Serve warm.

Nutritional Value (per serving):
- Calories: 200
- Carbohydrates: 40g
- Protein: 2g
- Fat: 6g
- Fiber: 5g

Cost per Serving:
Approximately $2.00

6. GRILLED LAMB CHOPS WITH ROSEMARY

History:
Lamb chops have been a delicacy in many cultures, particularly in Mediterranean and Middle Eastern cuisines. Grilling with rosemary adds a fragrant and flavourful touch, making this dish ideal for special occasions.

Ingredients:
- 4 lamb chops
- 2 tablespoons olive oil
- 2 cloves garlic, minced
- 1 tablespoon fresh rosemary, chopped
- Salt and pepper to taste

Possible Substitutes:
- Pork chops instead of lamb

Method of Preparation:
1. Preheat grill to medium-high heat.
2. In a small bowl, combine olive oil, garlic, rosemary, salt, and pepper.
3. Rub the mixture onto the lamb chops.
4. Grill lamb chops for 3-4 minutes per side for medium-rare, or until desired doneness.
5. Let rest for 5 minutes before serving.

Nutritional Value (per serving):
- Calories: 400
- Carbohydrates: 2g
- Protein: 25g
- Fat: 33g
- Fiber: 0g

Cost per Serving:
Approximately $6.00

7. QUINOA STUFFED MUSHROOMS

History:
Stuffed mushrooms have been a popular appetizer for centuries, with variations found in many cuisines. Using quinoa as a filling provides a nutritious and modern twist to this classic dish.

Ingredients:
- 12 large mushrooms, stems removed
- 1 cup cooked quinoa
- 1/4 cup grated Parmesan cheese
- 1/4 cup finely chopped spinach
- 2 cloves garlic, minced
- 2 tablespoons olive oil
- Salt and pepper to taste

Possible Substitutes:
- Brown rice instead of quinoa
- Feta cheese instead of Parmesan

Method of Preparation:
1. Preheat oven to 375°F (190°C).
2. In a bowl, combine cooked quinoa, Parmesan cheese, spinach, garlic, salt, and pepper.
3. Stuff the mixture into the mushroom

caps.
4. Place mushrooms on a baking sheet and drizzle with olive oil.
5. Bake for 15-20 minutes until mushrooms are tender and

filling is golden.
6. Serve hot.

Nutritional Value (per serving):
- Calories: 150
- Carbohydrates: 12g
- Protein: 6g
- Fat: 8g
- Fiber: 3g

Cost per Serving:
Approximately $2.50

8. BALSAMIC GLAZED BRUSSELS SPROUTS

History:
Brussels sprouts have been cultivated since ancient Rome and have gained popularity for their health benefits. Glazing with balsamic vinegar adds a sweet and tangy flavour, making them a delightful side dish for special occasions.

Ingredients:
- 1 lb Brussels sprouts, trimmed and halved
- 2 tablespoons olive oil
- 1/4 cup balsamic vinegar
- 1 tablespoon honey
- Salt and pepper to taste

Possible Substitutes:
- Broccoli or cauliflower instead of Brussels sprouts

Method of Preparation:
1. Preheat oven to 400°F (200°C).
2. Toss Brussels sprouts with olive oil, salt, and pepper.
3. Spread on a baking sheet and roast for 20-25 minutes until tender and crispy.
4. In a small saucepan, heat balsamic vinegar and honey until reduced by half.
5. Drizzle balsamic glaze over roasted Brussels sprouts.
6. Serve hot.

Nutritional Value (per serving):

- Calories: 150
- Carbohydrates: 18g
- Protein: 3g
- Fat: 8g
- Fiber: 4g

Cost per Serving:
Approximately $2.00

9. CAULIFLOWER MASH

History:
Cauliflower mash is a modern low-carb alternative to traditional mashed potatoes. It has gained popularity for its creamy texture and versatility in various cuisines.

Ingredients:
- 1 large head cauliflower, chopped
- 1/4 cup Greek yogurt
- 2 cloves garlic, minced
- 2 tablespoons butter
- Salt and pepper to taste

Possible Substitutes:
- Mashed turnips or parsnips for a different flavour

Method of Preparation:
1. Boil cauliflower in a large pot of salted water until tender, about 10 minutes.
2. Drain and transfer cauliflower to a food processor.
3. Add Greek yogurt, garlic, and butter, blending until smooth.
4. Season with salt and pepper to taste.
5. Serve hot.

Nutritional Value (per serving):
- Calories: 100
- Carbohydrates: 10g
- Protein: 3g

- Fat: 7g
- Fiber: 3g

Cost per Serving:
Approximately $1.50

10. ALMOND FLOUR CHOCOLATE CAKE

History:
Almond flour chocolate cake is a gluten-free dessert that has become popular in recent years. Made with almond flour, it offers a rich and moist texture while being suitable for those with dietary restrictions.

Ingredients:
- 1 1/2 cups almond flour
- 1/2 cup cocoa powder
- 1/2 cup coconut sugar
- 1/2 teaspoon baking soda
- 1/4 teaspoon salt
- 3 eggs
- 1/4 cup coconut oil, melted
- 1/4 cup almond milk
- 1 teaspoon vanilla extract

Possible Substitutes:
- Other nut flours like hazelnut or cashew
- Maple syrup instead of coconut sugar

Method of Preparation:
1. Preheat oven to 350°F (175°C).
2. In a large bowl, combine almond flour, cocoa powder, coconut sugar, baking soda, and salt.
3. In another bowl, whisk together eggs, coconut oil, almond milk, and vanilla extract.

4. Pour wet ingredients into dry ingredients and mix until well combined.
5. Pour batter into a greased 9-inch round cake pan.
6. Bake for 25-30 minutes until a toothpick inserted into the center comes out clean.
7. Let cool before serving.

Nutritional Value (per serving):
- Calories: 250
- Carbohydrates: 20g
- Protein: 7g
- Fat: 18g
- Fiber: 5g

Cost per Serving:
Approximately $3.00

Chapter 9: International Delights

1. SUSHI ROLLS WITH BROWN RICE

History:
Sushi originated in Japan and has become a beloved dish worldwide. Using brown rice adds a nutritional boost with more fibre and vitamins compared to traditional white rice.

Ingredients:
- 2 cups cooked brown rice
- 1/4 cup rice vinegar
- 2 tablespoons sugar
- 1 teaspoon salt
- 4 nori sheets
- 1 cucumber, julienned
- 1 avocado, sliced
- 1 carrot, julienned
- Soy sauce for serving

Possible Substitutes:
- Quinoa instead of brown rice
- Different vegetables like bell peppers or asparagus

Method of Preparation:
1. Mix rice vinegar, sugar, and salt into the cooked brown rice while it's still warm.
2. Lay a nori sheet on a bamboo sushi mat.
3. Spread a thin layer of brown rice over the nori, leaving a 1-inch border at the top.
4. Arrange cucumber, avocado, and carrot in a line across the

bottom of the nori.
5. Roll the sushi tightly using the bamboo mat.
6. Slice into bite-sized pieces and serve with soy sauce.

Nutritional Value (per serving):
- Calories: 300
- Carbohydrates: 50g
- Protein: 6g
- Fat: 10g
- Fiber: 7g

Cost per Serving:
Approximately $3.00

2. RATATOUILLE

History:
Ratatouille is a traditional French Provençal stewed vegetable dish originating from Nice. It is typically made with tomatoes, onions, zucchini, eggplant, and bell peppers.

Ingredients:
- 1 eggplant, diced
- 1 zucchini, diced
- 1 yellow squash, diced
- 1 red bell pepper, diced
- 1 yellow bell pepper, diced
- 1 onion, diced
- 2 cloves garlic, minced
- 4 tomatoes, diced
- 1/4 cup olive oil
- 1 teaspoon dried thyme
- 1 teaspoon dried basil
- Salt and pepper to taste

Possible Substitutes:
- Different herbs like rosemary or oregano
- Add mushrooms for extra flavour

Method of Preparation:
1. Preheat oven to 375°F (190°C).
2. In a large skillet, heat olive oil and sauté onion and garlic until soft.
3. Add eggplant, zucchini, squash, and bell peppers, cooking until slightly tender.

4. Stir in tomatoes, thyme, basil, salt, and pepper.

5. Transfer the mixture to a baking dish and bake for 30 minutes.

6. Serve hot or at room temperature.

Nutritional Value (per serving):
- Calories: 150
- Carbohydrates: 20g
- Protein: 3g
- Fat: 7g
- Fiber: 6g

Cost per Serving:
Approximately $2.50

3. TANDOORI CHICKEN

History:
Tandoori chicken is a popular Indian dish marinated in yogurt and spices, then roasted in a tandoor oven. It is known for its vibrant colour and rich flavour.

Ingredients:
- 4 chicken thighs
- 1 cup Greek yogurt
- 2 tablespoons lemon juice
- 2 tablespoons tandoori masala
- 1 teaspoon turmeric
- 1 teaspoon paprika
- 2 cloves garlic, minced
- 1-inch piece of ginger, grated
- Salt and pepper to taste

Possible Substitutes:
- Use tofu or tempeh for a vegetarian option
- Different spice blends for varied flavour

Method of Preparation:
1. In a large bowl, mix Greek yogurt, lemon juice, tandoori masala, turmeric, paprika, garlic, ginger, salt, and pepper.
2. Add chicken thighs and coat well with the marinade.
3. Cover and refrigerate for at least 4 hours or overnight.
4. Preheat oven to 400°F (200°C).
5. Place chicken on a baking sheet and bake for 25-30 minutes

until fully cooked.
6. Serve hot.

Nutritional Value (per serving):
- Calories: 350
- Carbohydrates: 10g
- Protein: 30g
- Fat: 20g
- Fiber: 2g

Cost per Serving:
Approximately $4.00

4. THAI GREEN CURRY WITH TOFU

History:
Thai green curry is a staple in Thai cuisine, known for its balance of spicy, sweet, and savoury flavours. This version uses tofu as a protein source, making it vegetarian-friendly.

Ingredients:
- 1 block firm tofu, cubed
- 1 can (14 oz) coconut milk
- 2 tablespoons green curry paste
- 1 cup green beans, trimmed
- 1 red bell pepper, sliced
- 1 zucchini, sliced
- 1 tablespoon soy sauce
- 1 tablespoon olive oil
- Fresh basil leaves for garnish

Possible Substitutes:
- Chicken or shrimp instead of tofu
- Different vegetables like broccoli or carrots

Method of Preparation:
1. Heat olive oil in a large skillet over medium heat.
2. Add green curry paste and cook for 1-2 minutes until fragrant.
3. Stir in coconut milk and bring to a simmer.
4. Add tofu, green beans, bell pepper, zucchini, and soy sauce.
5. Simmer for 10-15 minutes until vegetables are tender.
6. Garnish with fresh basil leaves and serve hot.

Nutritional Value (per serving):
- Calories: 300
- Carbohydrates: 20g
- Protein: 15g
- Fat: 20g
- Fiber: 5g

Cost per Serving:
Approximately $3.50

5. MOROCCAN CHICKPEA STEW

History:
Moroccan cuisine is known for its rich and aromatic flavours.
This chickpea stew is a traditional dish that combines a variety
of spices to create a hearty and nutritious meal.

Ingredients:
- 1 can (15 oz) chickpeas, drained and rinsed
- 1 onion, diced
- 2 cloves garlic, minced
- 1 carrot, diced
- 1 zucchini, diced
- 1 can (14.5 oz) diced tomatoes
- 2 cups vegetable broth
- 1 teaspoon cumin
- 1 teaspoon paprika
- 1/2 teaspoon cinnamon
- 1/2 teaspoon turmeric
- 2 tablespoons olive oil
- Salt and pepper to taste

Possible Substitutes:
- Different beans like lentils or black beans
- Add raisins or dried apricots for sweetness

Method of Preparation:
1. Heat olive oil in a large pot over medium heat.
2. Add onion, garlic, carrot, and zucchini, cooking until

softened.

3. Stir in chickpeas, diced tomatoes, vegetable broth, cumin, paprika, cinnamon, turmeric, salt, and pepper.

4. Bring to a boil, then reduce heat and simmer for 20-25 minutes until vegetables are tender.

5. Serve hot.

Nutritional Value (per serving):
- Calories: 250
- Carbohydrates: 35g
- Protein: 8g
- Fat: 8g
- Fiber: 10g

Cost per Serving:
Approximately $2.50

6. SPANISH GAZPACHO

History:
Gazpacho is a cold soup from Spain, traditionally made with tomatoes, peppers, cucumbers, and onions. It is particularly popular in the summer months due to its refreshing qualities.

Ingredients:
- 4 large tomatoes, chopped
- 1 cucumber, peeled and chopped
- 1 red bell pepper, chopped
- 1 green bell pepper, chopped
- 1 small red onion, chopped
- 2 cloves garlic, minced
- 3 cups tomato juice
- 1/4 cup olive oil
- 2 tablespoons red wine vinegar
- Salt and pepper to taste

Possible Substitutes:
- Use different colors of bell peppers for variety
- Add bread for a thicker consistency

Method of Preparation:
1. In a blender, combine tomatoes, cucumber, red bell pepper, green bell pepper, red onion, garlic, tomato juice, olive oil, red wine vinegar, salt, and pepper.
2. Blend until smooth.
3. Chill in the refrigerator for at least 2 hours before serving.

4. Serve cold.

Nutritional Value (per serving):
- Calories: 150
- Carbohydrates: 20g
- Protein: 3g
- Fat: 8g
- Fiber: 5g

Cost per Serving:
Approximately $2.00

7. ITALIAN CAPRESE SALAD

History:
Caprese salad is a simple Italian dish named after the island of Capri. It features fresh tomatoes, mozzarella, and basil, drizzled with olive oil and balsamic vinegar.

Ingredients:
- 4 large tomatoes, sliced
- 1 ball fresh mozzarella, sliced
- 1/4 cup fresh basil leaves
- 2 tablespoons olive oil
- 1 tablespoon balsamic vinegar
- Salt and pepper to taste

Possible Substitutes:
- Use heirloom tomatoes for different flavours and colours
- Add avocado for extra creaminess

Method of Preparation:
1. Arrange tomato slices, mozzarella slices, and basil leaves on a serving platter.
2. Drizzle with olive oil and balsamic

vinegar.
3. Season with salt and pepper.
4. Serve immediately.

Nutritional Value (per serving):
- Calories: 200

- Carbohydrates: 7g
- Protein: 10g
- Fat: 15g
- Fiber: 2g

Cost per Serving:
Approximately $3.00

8. VIETNAMESE SPRING ROLLS

History:
Vietnamese spring rolls, also known as "gỏi cuốn," are fresh, light, and healthy. They are typically filled with shrimp, vegetables, and herbs, wrapped in rice paper.

Ingredients:
- 8 rice paper wrappers
- 1/2 lb cooked shrimp, sliced in half lengthwise
- 1 cup shredded lettuce
- 1 cup shredded carrots
- 1/2 cup fresh mint leaves
- 1/2 cup fresh cilantro leaves
- 1/2 cup vermicelli noodles, cooked

Possible Substitutes:
- Use tofu instead of shrimp for a vegetarian version
- Different herbs like basil

Method of Preparation:
1. Dip each rice paper wrapper in warm water for a few seconds to soften.
2. Lay the wrapper flat and place shrimp, lettuce, carrots, mint, cilantro, and vermicelli noodles in the center.
3. Fold in the sides and roll tightly.
4. Serve with a dipping sauce like hoisin or peanut sauce.

Nutritional Value (per serving):

- Calories: 150
- Carbohydrates: 20g
- Protein: 10g
- Fat: 2g
- Fiber: 3g

Cost per Serving:
Approximately $2.50

9. MEXICAN QUINOA BOWL

History:
Quinoa bowls have become a popular way to combine grains, vegetables, and proteins in a nutritious meal. This Mexican-inspired version includes black beans, corn, avocado, and a zesty lime dressing.

Ingredients:
- 1 cup cooked quinoa
- 1 can (15 oz) black beans, drained and rinsed
- 1 cup corn kernels
- 1 avocado, diced
- 1/2 cup cherry tomatoes, halved
- 1/4 cup red onion, diced
- 1/4 cup fresh cilantro, chopped
- 2 tablespoons olive oil
- 2 tablespoons lime juice
- Salt and pepper to taste

Possible Substitutes:
- Use brown rice instead of quinoa
- Add different vegetables like bell peppers

Method of Preparation:
1. In a large bowl, combine cooked quinoa, black beans, corn, avocado, cherry tomatoes, red onion, and cilantro.
2. In a small bowl, whisk together olive oil, lime juice, salt, and pepper.

3. Pour dressing over the quinoa mixture and toss to combine.
4. Serve immediately or refrigerate until ready to serve.

Nutritional Value (per serving):
- Calories: 300
- Carbohydrates: 40g
- Protein: 10g
- Fat: 15g
- Fiber: 10g

Cost per Serving:
Approximately $3.00

10. MIDDLE EASTERN TABOULEH

History:
Tabouleh is a traditional Middle Eastern salad made with parsley, mint, tomatoes, and bulgur wheat. It is known for its fresh flavours and nutritional benefits.

Ingredients:
- 1 cup bulgur wheat
- 2 cups boiling water
- 1 cup fresh parsley, chopped
- 1/2 cup fresh mint, chopped
- 4 tomatoes, diced
- 1 cucumber, diced
- 1/4 cup red onion, diced
- 1/4 cup olive oil
- 1/4 cup lemon juice
- Salt and pepper to taste

Possible Substitutes:
- Use quinoa instead of bulgur wheat for a gluten-free option

Method of Preparation:
1. Place bulgur wheat in a large bowl and pour boiling water over it. Cover and let sit for 20 minutes, then drain any excess water.
2. Add parsley, mint, tomatoes, cucumber, and red onion to the bulgur.
3. In a small bowl, whisk together olive oil, lemon juice, salt, and pepper.

4. Pour dressing over the salad and toss to combine.
5. Serve immediately or refrigerate until ready to serve.

Nutritional Value (per serving):
- Calories: 180
- Carbohydrates: 30g
- Protein: 4g
- Fat: 7g
- Fiber: 6g

Cost per Serving:
Approximately $2.00

Chapter 10: Desserts

1. DARK CHOCOLATE AVOCADO MOUSSE

History:
Dark chocolate mousse has been a classic French dessert for centuries. This version uses avocado for a creamy texture and added nutritional benefits, creating a healthier twist on the traditional recipe.

Ingredients:
- 2 ripe avocados
- 1/2 cup dark chocolate, melted
- 1/4 cup cocoa powder
- 1/4 cup honey or maple syrup
- 1 teaspoon vanilla extract
- Pinch of salt

Possible Substitutes:
- Agave nectar instead of honey
- Carob powder instead of cocoa powder

Method of Preparation:
1. In a food processor, blend avocados until smooth.
2. Add melted dark chocolate, cocoa powder, honey or maple syrup, vanilla extract, and salt.
3. Blend until well combined and smooth.
4. Spoon mousse into serving dishes and refrigerate for at least 30 minutes before serving.

Nutritional Value (per serving):

- Calories: 250
- Carbohydrates: 25g
- Protein: 3g
- Fat: 18g
- Fiber: 7g

Cost per Serving:
Approximately $3.00

2. BERRY PARFAIT

History:
Parfaits are a layered dessert that originated in France. This berry parfait combines Greek yogurt with fresh berries for a light and nutritious treat.

Ingredients:
- 1 cup Greek yogurt
- 1/2 cup mixed berries (strawberries, blueberries, raspberries)
- 1/4 cup granola
- 1 tablespoon honey

Possible Substitutes:
- Plant-based yogurt for a dairy-free option
- Any seasonal fruits instead of berries

Method of Preparation:
1. In a serving glass, layer Greek yogurt, mixed berries, and granola.
2. Drizzle with honey.
3. Repeat layers as desired.
4. Serve immediately.

Nutritional Value (per serving):
- Calories: 200
- Carbohydrates: 30g
- Protein: 10g
- Fat: 6g
- Fiber: 4g

Cost per Serving:

Approximately $2.50

3. ALMOND FLOUR COOKIES

History:
Almond flour cookies have become popular in recent years, especially among those following gluten-free diets. These cookies are simple to make and provide a delightful nutty flavour.

Ingredients:
- 2 cups almond flour
- 1/4 cup coconut oil, melted
- 1/4 cup honey or maple syrup
- 1 teaspoon vanilla extract
- 1/2 teaspoon baking soda
- Pinch of salt

Possible Substitutes:
- Agave nectar instead of honey
- Any nut or seed butter for added flavour

Method of Preparation:
1. Preheat oven to 350°F (175°C).
2. In a bowl, mix almond flour, coconut oil, honey or maple syrup, vanilla extract, baking soda, and salt until well combined.
3. Scoop tablespoon-sized portions of dough onto a baking sheet lined with parchment paper.
4. Flatten each cookie slightly with the back of a spoon.
5. Bake for 10-12 minutes until edges are golden brown.
6. Let cool before serving.

Nutritional Value (per serving):
- Calories: 150
- Carbohydrates: 8g
- Protein: 4g
- Fat: 12g
- Fiber: 3g

Cost per Serving:
Approximately $2.00

4. COCONUT MACAROONS

History:
Coconut macaroons are a traditional sweet treat found in many cultures. These cookies are made primarily of coconut, providing a chewy texture and rich flavour.

Ingredients:
- 2 cups shredded coconut
- 1/2 cup sweetened condensed milk
- 1 teaspoon vanilla extract
- 1/4 teaspoon salt

Possible Substitutes:
- Coconut cream instead of sweetened condensed milk for a dairy-free option

Method of Preparation:
1. Preheat oven to 350°F (175°C).
2. In a bowl, mix shredded coconut, sweetened condensed milk, vanilla extract, and salt until well combined.
3. Scoop tablespoon-sized portions of mixture onto a baking sheet lined with parchment paper.
4. Bake for 15-20 minutes until golden brown.
5. Let cool before serving.

Nutritional Value (per serving):
- Calories: 120
- Carbohydrates: 14g

- Protein: 2g
- Fat: 7g
- Fiber: 3g

Cost per Serving:
Approximately $2.00

5. LEMON CHIA SEED MUFFINS

History:
Lemon chia seed muffins combine the refreshing flavour of lemon with the nutritional benefits of chia seeds. These muffins are perfect for a light dessert or snack.

Ingredients:
- 2 cups almond flour
- 1/4 cup chia seeds
- 1/4 cup honey or maple syrup
- 1/2 cup almond milk
- 2 eggs
- 1/4 cup coconut oil, melted
- 1 teaspoon baking soda
- 1 teaspoon vanilla extract
- Zest and juice of 1 lemon

Possible Substitutes:
- Flaxseed meal instead of chia seeds
- Agave nectar instead of honey

Method of Preparation:
1. Preheat oven to 350°F (175°C).
2. In a bowl, mix almond flour, chia seeds, honey or maple syrup, almond milk, eggs, coconut oil, baking soda, vanilla extract, lemon zest, and lemon juice until well combined.
3. Scoop batter into a lined muffin tin.
4. Bake for 20-25 minutes until a toothpick inserted into the

center comes out clean.
5. Let cool before serving.

Nutritional Value (per serving):
- Calories: 200
- Carbohydrates: 15g
- Protein: 6g
- Fat: 14g
- Fiber: 5g

Cost per Serving:
Approximately $2.50

6. BAKED PEARS WITH CINNAMON

History:
Baked pears are a simple and elegant dessert that highlights the natural sweetness of the fruit. This dish is often enjoyed during the fall and winter months.

Ingredients:
- 4 pears, halved and cored
- 2 tablespoons honey
- 1 teaspoon cinnamon
- 1/4 cup chopped walnuts

Possible Substitutes:
- Apples instead of pears
- Pecans or almonds instead of walnuts

Method of Preparation:
1. Preheat oven to 350°F (175°C).
2. Place pear halves in a baking dish.
3. Drizzle with honey and sprinkle with cinnamon.
4. Top with chopped walnuts.
5. Bake for 25-30 minutes until pears are tender.
6. Serve warm.

Nutritional Value (per serving):
- Calories: 150
- Carbohydrates: 25g
- Protein: 2g

- Fat: 5g
- Fiber: 5g

Cost per Serving:
Approximately $2.00

7. RICOTTA CHEESE WITH BERRIES

History:
Ricotta cheese has been used in Italian cuisine for centuries. Pairing it with fresh berries creates a light and refreshing dessert that is both nutritious and delicious.

Ingredients:
- 1 cup ricotta cheese
- 1/2 cup mixed berries (strawberries, blueberries, raspberries)
- 1 tablespoon honey
- 1 teaspoon lemon zest

Possible Substitutes:
- Greek yogurt instead of ricotta cheese
- Any seasonal fruits instead of berries

Method of Preparation:
1. In a bowl, mix ricotta cheese, honey, and lemon zest until smooth.
2. Spoon ricotta mixture into serving bowls.
3. Top with mixed berries.
4. Serve immediately.

Nutritional Value (per serving):
- Calories: 200
- Carbohydrates: 15g
- Protein: 10g
- Fat: 12g

- Fiber: 3g

Cost per Serving: Approximately $2.50

8. FROZEN YOGURT BARK

History:
Frozen yogurt bark is a modern dessert that combines the creamy texture of yogurt with the crunch of nuts and fruits. It is a healthy and refreshing treat for hot days.

Ingredients:
- 2 cups Greek yogurt
- 1/4 cup honey
- 1/2 cup mixed berries
- 1/4 cup chopped nuts (almonds, walnuts, pistachios)

Possible Substitutes:
- Plant-based yogurt for a dairy-free option
- Any dried fruits or seeds

Method of Preparation:
1. In a bowl, mix Greek yogurt and honey until well combined.
2. Spread the yogurt mixture evenly on a baking sheet lined with parchment paper.
3. Sprinkle with mixed berries and chopped nuts.
4. Freeze for at least 2 hours until solid.
5. Break into pieces and serve.

Nutritional Value (per serving):
- Calories: 150
- Carbohydrates: 20g
- Protein: 8g

- Fat: 6g
- Fiber: 2g

Cost per Serving:
Approximately $2.00

9. CHIA SEED JAM

History:
Chia seed jam is a healthier alternative to traditional jam, using chia seeds as a natural thickener. It is easy to make and

can be used in various desserts or as a spread.

Ingredients:
- 2 cups fresh or frozen berries
- 2 tablespoons chia seeds
- 1-2 tablespoons honey or maple syrup
- 1 teaspoon lemon juice

Possible Substitutes:
- Any fruits of choice

Method of Preparation:
1. In a saucepan, heat berries over medium heat until they begin to break down.
2. Mash the berries with a fork or potato masher.
3. Stir in chia seeds, honey or maple syrup, and lemon juice.
4. Cook for 5-10 minutes until the mixture thickens.
5. Let cool before serving.

Nutritional Value (per serving):
- Calories: 50
- Carbohydrates: 10g
- Protein: 1g
- Fat: 1g
- Fiber: 3g

Cost per Serving:

Approximately $1.50

10. OATMEAL RAISIN COOKIES

History:
Oatmeal raisin cookies are a classic American treat, known for their chewy texture and sweet flavour. These cookies are a healthier option compared to many other desserts.

Ingredients:
- 1 cup rolled oats
- 1/2 cup almond flour
- 1/2 cup raisins
- 1/4 cup coconut oil, melted
- 1/4 cup honey or maple syrup
- 1 teaspoon vanilla extract
- 1/2 teaspoon cinnamon
- 1/4 teaspoon baking soda
- Pinch of salt

Possible Substitutes:
- Dried cranberries instead of raisins
- Any nut butter for added flavour

Method of Preparation:
1. Preheat oven to 350°F (175°C).
2. In a bowl, mix rolled oats, almond flour, raisins, coconut oil, honey or maple syrup, vanilla extract, cinnamon, baking soda, and salt until well combined.
3. Scoop tablespoon-sized portions of dough onto a baking sheet lined with parchment paper.

4. Flatten each cookie slightly with the back of a spoon.
5. Bake for 10-12 minutes until edges are golden brown.
6. Let cool before serving.

Nutritional Value (per serving):
- Calories: 120
- Carbohydrates: 18g
- Protein: 2g
- Fat: 5g
- Fiber: 3g

Cost per Serving:
Approximately $1.50

Chapter 11: Low-Carb Favourites

1. ZUCCHINI PIZZA BOATS

History:
Zucchini pizza boats offer a low-carb alternative to traditional pizza, utilizing zucchini as the base. This dish is part of the growing trend of using vegetables in innovative ways to create healthier versions of favourite foods.

Ingredients:
- 4 medium zucchinis, halved lengthwise and seeds scooped out
- 1 cup marinara sauce
- 1 cup shredded mozzarella cheese
- 1/2 cup mini pepperoni slices
- 1/4 cup grated Parmesan cheese
- 1 tablespoon olive oil
- Salt and pepper to taste

Possible Substitutes:
- Different cheeses like cheddar or feta
- Various toppings like mushrooms, bell peppers, or olives

Method of Preparation:
1. Preheat oven to 375°F (190°C).
2. Brush zucchini halves with olive oil and season with salt and pepper.
3. Place zucchini halves on a baking sheet.
4. Spoon marinara sauce into each zucchini half.
5. Sprinkle with mozzarella cheese, mini pepperoni slices, and Parmesan cheese.

6. Bake for 20-25 minutes until the cheese is bubbly and golden.
7. Serve hot.

Nutritional Value (per serving):
- Calories: 200
- Carbohydrates: 6g
- Protein: 12g
- Fat: 14g
- Fiber: 2g

Cost per Serving:
Approximately $2.50

2. CAULIFLOWER FRIED RICE

History:
Cauliflower fried rice has become popular as a low-carb substitute for traditional fried rice. This dish mimics the texture of rice while providing additional nutrients from the cauliflower.

Ingredients:
- 1 head cauliflower, grated into rice-sized pieces
- 1 cup mixed vegetables (peas, carrots, bell peppers)
- 2 eggs, beaten
- 2 tablespoons soy sauce
- 1 tablespoon olive oil
- 2 cloves garlic, minced
- 1 teaspoon grated ginger
- Salt and pepper to taste

Possible Substitutes:
- Broccoli rice instead of cauliflower rice
- Tamari for a gluten-free option

Method of Preparation:
1. Heat olive oil in a large skillet over medium-high heat.
2. Add garlic and ginger, cooking for 1 minute.
3. Add mixed vegetables and stir-fry for 5-7 minutes until tender.
4. Push vegetables to one side of the skillet and pour beaten eggs into the other side, scrambling them.

5. Add grated cauliflower and soy sauce, stirring to combine.
6. Cook for another 3-5 minutes until cauliflower is tender.
7. Season with salt and pepper to taste and serve hot.

Nutritional Value (per serving):
- Calories: 150
- Carbohydrates: 10g
- Protein: 8g
- Fat: 10g
- Fiber: 4g

Cost per Serving:
Approximately $2.00

3. CHICKEN LETTUCE WRAPS

History:
Lettuce wraps are a low-carb alternative to traditional wraps and have roots in Asian cuisine. This dish uses lettuce leaves to encase a flavourful chicken filling.

Ingredients:
- 1 lb ground chicken
- 1 cup water chestnuts, diced
- 1/2 cup green onions, sliced
- 1/4 cup hoisin sauce
- 2 tablespoons soy sauce
- 1 tablespoon rice vinegar
- 1 tablespoon olive oil
- 2 cloves garlic, minced
- 1 head butter lettuce, leaves separated

Possible Substitutes:
- Ground turkey instead of chicken
- Different vegetables like bell peppers or mushrooms

Method of Preparation:
1. Heat olive oil in a large skillet over medium-high heat.
2. Add garlic and cook for 1 minute until fragrant.
3. Add ground chicken and cook until browned.
4. Stir in water chestnuts, green onions, hoisin sauce, soy sauce, and rice vinegar.
5. Cook for another 2-3 minutes until heated through.

6. Spoon chicken mixture into lettuce leaves.
7. Serve immediately.

Nutritional Value (per serving):
- Calories: 250
- Carbohydrates: 12g
- Protein: 20g
- Fat: 14g
- Fiber: 3g

Cost per Serving:
Approximately $3.00

4. EGG MUFFINS WITH VEGGIES

History:
Egg muffins are a convenient, portable, and low-carb breakfast option. These muffins are packed with protein and vegetables, making them a nutritious start to the day.

Ingredients:
- 6 large eggs
- 1/2 cup spinach, chopped
- 1/2 cup bell peppers, diced
- 1/4 cup red onion, diced
- 1/4 cup shredded cheese
- 1/4 cup milk (optional)
- Salt and pepper to taste

Possible Substitutes:
- Any preferred vegetables like mushrooms or tomatoes
- Dairy-free milk for a lactose-free option

Method of Preparation:
1. Preheat oven to 350°F (175°C).
2. In a large bowl, whisk together eggs, milk (if using), salt, and pepper.
3. Stir in spinach, bell peppers, red onion, and cheese.
4. Pour the egg mixture into a greased muffin tin, filling each cup about 3/4 full.
5. Bake for 20-25 minutes until the eggs are set and golden.
6. Let cool before removing from the tin.

7. Serve warm or store in the refrigerator for up to 3 days.

Nutritional Value (per serving):
- Calories: 100
- Carbohydrates: 2g
- Protein: 8g
- Fat: 7g
- Fiber: 1g

Cost per Serving:
Approximately $1.50

5. SPAGHETTI SQUASH WITH MARINARA

History:
Spaghetti squash is a low-carb alternative to pasta, with a stringy texture that resembles spaghetti when cooked. This dish pairs the squash with marinara sauce for a healthy and satisfying meal.

Ingredients:
- 1 large spaghetti squash
- 2 cups marinara sauce
- 1/4 cup grated Parmesan cheese
- 2 tablespoons olive oil
- Salt and pepper to taste

Possible Substitutes:
- Different sauces like pesto or Alfredo
- Zucchini noodles instead of spaghetti squash

Method of Preparation:
1. Preheat oven to 375°F (190°C).
2. Cut the spaghetti squash in half lengthwise and scoop out the seeds.
3. Brush the inside of the squash with olive oil and season with salt and pepper.
4. Place the squash halves cut side down on a baking sheet.

5. Bake for 40-45 minutes until tender.

6. Use a fork to scrape out the strands of squash.

7. Heat marinara sauce in a saucepan over medium heat.

8. Serve spaghetti squash topped with marinara sauce and grated Parmesan cheese.

Nutritional Value (per serving):
- Calories: 150
- Carbohydrates: 20g
- Protein: 4g
- Fat: 7g
- Fiber: 4g

Cost per Serving:
Approximately $2.50

6. SHRIMP SCAMPI WITH ZOODLES

History:
Shrimp scampi is a classic Italian-American dish, traditionally served over pasta. Using zucchini noodles (zoodles) instead of pasta creates a low-carb version that is equally delicious.

Ingredients:
- 1 lb large shrimp, peeled and deveined
- 4 medium zucchinis, spiralized
- 4 cloves garlic, minced
- 1/4 cup white wine (optional)
- 1/4 cup chicken broth
- 2 tablespoons lemon juice
- 1/4 cup Parmesan cheese, grated
- 2 tablespoons olive oil
- Salt and pepper to taste
- Fresh parsley for garnish

Possible Substitutes:
- Chicken instead of shrimp
- Vegetable broth instead of chicken broth

Method of Preparation:
1. Heat olive oil in a large skillet over medium-high heat.
2. Add garlic and cook for 1 minute until fragrant.
3. Add shrimp and cook until pink and opaque.
4. Remove shrimp from the skillet and set aside.
5. In the same skillet, add white wine (if using), chicken broth,

and lemon juice.
6. Bring to a simmer and cook for 2-3 minutes.
7. Add zucchini noodles and cook for 2-3 minutes until tender.
8. Return shrimp to the skillet and toss to combine.
9. Season with salt and pepper.
10. Serve topped with Parmesan cheese and fresh parsley.

Nutritional Value (per serving):
- Calories: 250
- Carbohydrates: 6g
- Protein: 30g
- Fat: 12g
- Fiber: 2g

Cost per Serving:
Approximately $4.00

7. BROCCOLI AND CHEESE CASSEROLE

History:
Broccoli and cheese casserole is a comforting dish that combines tender broccoli with creamy cheese sauce. This low-carb version uses fewer carbs while maintaining the rich flavours.

Ingredients:
- 4 cups broccoli florets
- 1 cup shredded cheddar cheese
- 1/2 cup Greek yogurt
- 1/4 cup grated Parmesan cheese
- 2 cloves garlic, minced
- 1/4 cup almond flour
- 1 tablespoon olive oil
- Salt and pepper to taste

Possible Substitutes:
- Cauliflower instead of broccoli
- Any preferred cheese like mozzarella or Swiss

Method of Preparation:
1. Preheat oven to 375°F (190°C).
2. Steam broccoli florets until tender.
3. In a large bowl, combine steamed broccoli, cheddar cheese, Greek yogurt, garlic, salt, and pepper.
4. Transfer the mixture to a greased baking dish.
5. In a small bowl, mix almond flour, Parmesan cheese, and olive

oil.
6. Sprinkle the almond flour mixture over the broccoli.
7. Bake for 20-25 minutes until the top is golden brown and bubbly.
8. Serve hot.

Nutritional Value (per serving):
- Calories: 200
- Carbohydrates: 10g
- Protein: 10g
- Fat: 14g
- Fiber: 4g

Cost per Serving:
Approximately $3.00

8. BUFFALO CAULIFLOWER BITES

History:
Buffalo cauliflower bites are a vegetarian alternative to buffalo wings, providing the same spicy kick with a healthier twist. These bites are perfect for appetizers or snacks.

Ingredients:
- 1 head cauliflower, cut into bite-sized florets
- 1/2 cup almond flour
- 1/2 cup water
- 1/2 cup buffalo sauce
- 2 tablespoons olive oil
- 1 teaspoon garlic powder
- 1 teaspoon onion powder
- Salt and pepper to taste

Possible Substitutes:
- Different hot sauces for varied flavours
- Any other vegetables like broccoli or Brussels sprouts

Method of Preparation:
1. Preheat oven to 450°F (230°C).
2. In a large bowl, mix almond flour, water, garlic powder, onion powder, salt, and pepper to form a batter.
3. Dip cauliflower florets into the batter, ensuring they are well coated.
4. Place coated cauliflower on a baking sheet lined with parchment paper.

5. Bake for 20-25 minutes until crispy.
6. In a large bowl, toss baked cauliflower with buffalo sauce and olive oil.
7. Return to the baking sheet and bake for another 10 minutes.
8. Serve hot with celery sticks and ranch or blue cheese dressing.

Nutritional Value (per serving):
- Calories: 150
- Carbohydrates: 10g
- Protein: 3g
- Fat: 10g
- Fiber: 3g

Cost per Serving:
Approximately $2.50

9. SPINACH AND MUSHROOM FRITTATA

History:
A frittata is an Italian egg-based dish similar to an omelette or quiche. This version includes spinach and mushrooms, making it a nutritious and low-carb meal.

Ingredients:
- 8 large eggs
- 1 cup spinach, chopped
- 1 cup mushrooms, sliced
- 1/2 cup shredded cheese
- 1/4 cup milk (optional)
- 1 tablespoon olive oil
- 2 cloves garlic, minced
- Salt and pepper to taste

Possible Substitutes:
- Any preferred vegetables like bell peppers or tomatoes
- Dairy-free milk for a lactose-free option

Method of Preparation:
1. Preheat oven to 375°F (190°C).
2. Heat olive oil in an oven-safe skillet over medium heat.
3. Add garlic and mushrooms, cooking until mushrooms are tender.

4. Stir in spinach and cook until wilted.
5. In a bowl, whisk together eggs, milk (if using), salt, and pepper.
6. Pour the egg mixture into the skillet and sprinkle with shredded cheese.
7. Cook on the stovetop for 2-3 minutes until the edges start to set.
8. Transfer the skillet to the oven and bake for 10-12 minutes until the eggs are fully set.
9. Let cool slightly before slicing and serving.

Nutritional Value (per serving):
- Calories: 200
- Carbohydrates: 3g
- Protein: 14g
- Fat: 15g
- Fiber: 1g

Cost per Serving:
Approximately $2.50

10. BEEF AND BROCCOLI STIR-FRY

History:
Beef and broccoli stir-fry is a classic Chinese-American dish known for its savoury flavours and quick preparation. This low-carb version is packed with protein and vegetables.

Ingredients:
- 1 lb beef sirloin, sliced thinly
- 3 cups broccoli florets
- 2 tablespoons soy sauce
- 1 tablespoon oyster sauce
- 1 tablespoon olive oil
- 2 cloves garlic, minced
- 1 teaspoon grated ginger
- 1/4 cup beef broth
- Salt and pepper to taste

Possible Substitutes:
- Chicken or tofu instead of beef
- Tamari for a gluten-free option

Method of Preparation:
1. Heat olive oil in a large skillet over medium-high heat.
2. Add garlic and ginger, cooking for 1 minute until fragrant.
3. Add beef slices and cook until browned.
4. Remove beef from the skillet and set aside.
5. In the same skillet, add broccoli and beef broth, cooking until broccoli is tender.

6. Return beef to the skillet and stir in soy sauce and oyster sauce.

7. Cook for another 2-3 minutes until everything is heated through.

8. Season with salt and pepper to taste and serve hot.

Nutritional Value (per serving):
- Calories: 300
- Carbohydrates: 10g
- Protein: 25g
- Fat: 18g
- Fiber: 4g

Cost per Serving:
Approximately $4.00

Chapter 12: Quick and Easy

1. CHICKEN AND VEGGIE SKEWERS

History:
Skewers, or kebabs, have been a part of Middle Eastern and Mediterranean cuisine for centuries. This quick and easy dish combines marinated chicken with fresh vegetables, making it a perfect option for a healthy meal.

Ingredients:
- 2 chicken breasts, cut into cubes
- 1 red bell pepper, cut into chunks
- 1 yellow bell pepper, cut into chunks
- 1 zucchini, sliced
- 1 red onion, cut into chunks
- 2 tablespoons olive oil
- 2 tablespoons lemon juice
- 1 teaspoon dried oregano
- Salt and pepper to taste
- Wooden or metal skewers

Possible Substitutes:
- Tofu or shrimp instead of chicken
- Any preferred vegetables like cherry tomatoes or mushrooms

Method of Preparation:
1. In a large bowl, mix olive oil, lemon juice, oregano, salt, and pepper.
2. Add chicken cubes and marinate for at least 30 minutes.
3. Preheat grill to medium-high heat.

4. Thread chicken and vegetables onto skewers.
5. Grill skewers for 10-12 minutes, turning occasionally, until chicken is fully cooked.
6. Serve hot.

Nutritional Value (per serving):
- Calories: 250
- Carbohydrates: 8g
- Protein: 25g
- Fat: 12g
- Fiber: 3g

Cost per Serving:
Approximately $3.00

2. AVOCADO AND TUNA SALAD

History:
Avocado and tuna salad is a modern, healthy dish that combines creamy avocado with protein-rich tuna. It is quick to prepare and packed with nutrients.

Ingredients:
- 1 avocado, diced
- 1 can (5 oz) tuna, drained
- 1/4 cup red onion, finely chopped
- 1 tablespoon lemon juice
- 1 tablespoon olive oil
- Salt and pepper to taste

Possible Substitutes:
- Salmon instead of tuna
- Different vegetables like cherry tomatoes or cucumber

Method of Preparation:
1. In a bowl, combine diced avocado, tuna, and red onion.
2. Drizzle with lemon juice and olive oil.
3. Season with salt and pepper.
4. Mix gently to combine.
5. Serve immediately.

Nutritional Value (per serving):
- Calories: 300
- Carbohydrates: 10g

- Protein: 20g
- Fat: 22g
- Fiber: 7g

Cost per Serving:
Approximately $2.50

3. SPICY CHICKPEA SALAD

History:

Chickpeas have been a staple in Mediterranean and Middle Eastern diets for thousands of years. This spicy chickpea salad is quick to make and offers a flavourful and nutritious meal.

Ingredients:
- 1 can (15 oz) chickpeas, drained and rinsed
- 1/2 cup cherry tomatoes, halved
- 1/4 cup red onion, finely chopped
- 1/4 cup fresh cilantro, chopped
- 1 tablespoon olive oil
- 1 tablespoon lemon juice
- 1 teaspoon ground cumin
- 1/2 teaspoon paprika
- 1/4 teaspoon cayenne pepper (optional)
- Salt and pepper to taste

Possible Substitutes:
- Black beans or white beans instead of chickpeas
- Different herbs like parsley or mint

Method of Preparation:
1. In a large bowl, combine chickpeas, cherry tomatoes, red onion, and cilantro.
2. In a small bowl, whisk together olive oil, lemon juice, cumin, paprika, cayenne pepper, salt, and pepper.
3. Pour the dressing over the chickpea mixture and toss to

combine.

4. Serve immediately or refrigerate until ready to serve.

Nutritional Value (per serving):
- Calories: 200
- Carbohydrates: 28g
- Protein: 6g
- Fat: 8g
- Fiber: 8g

Cost per Serving:
Approximately $1.50

4. BAKED CHICKEN WINGS

History:
Chicken wings have been a favourite appetizer and party food in American cuisine for decades. Baking them provides a healthier alternative to frying.

Ingredients:
- 2 lbs chicken wings
- 1/4 cup olive oil
- 1 teaspoon garlic powder
- 1 teaspoon paprika
- 1 teaspoon salt
- 1/2 teaspoon black pepper

Possible Substitutes:
- Use drumsticks or chicken thighs
- Different seasonings like Cajun spice or lemon pepper

Method of Preparation:
1. Preheat oven to 400°F (200°C).
2. In a large bowl, mix olive oil, garlic powder, paprika, salt, and pepper.
3. Add chicken wings and toss to coat evenly.
4. Arrange wings on a baking sheet lined with parchment paper.
5. Bake for 40-45 minutes, turning halfway, until crispy and fully cooked.
6. Serve hot.

Nutritional Value (per serving):
- Calories: 300
- Carbohydrates: 0g
- Protein: 20g
- Fat: 24g
- Fiber: 0g

Cost per Serving:
Approximately $3.50

5. TOMATO BASIL SOUP

History:
Tomato basil soup is a classic comfort food with roots in Italian cuisine. It is known for its simplicity and rich flavour, making it a popular quick and easy meal.

Ingredients:
- 4 cups diced tomatoes (fresh or canned)
- 1 cup vegetable broth
- 1/2 cup chopped fresh basil
- 1/2 cup diced onion
- 2 cloves garlic, minced
- 1 tablespoon olive oil
- Salt and pepper to taste

Possible Substitutes:
- Use chicken broth instead of vegetable broth
- Add cream for a creamier texture

Method of Preparation:
1. Heat olive oil in a large pot over medium heat.
2. Add onion and garlic, cooking until soft.
3. Stir in diced tomatoes and vegetable broth.
4. Bring to a boil, then reduce heat and simmer for 15-20 minutes.
5. Use an immersion blender to puree the soup until smooth.
6. Stir in fresh basil and season with salt and pepper.
7. Serve hot.

Nutritional Value (per serving):
- Calories: 150
- Carbohydrates: 20g
- Protein: 3g
- Fat: 7g
- Fiber: 4g

Cost per Serving:
Approximately $2.00

6. VEGGIE QUESADILLA

History:
Quesadillas are a staple in Mexican cuisine, traditionally made with cheese and tortillas. This veggie version is quick to make and loaded with nutritious vegetables.

Ingredients:
- 2 whole wheat tortillas
- 1/2 cup shredded cheese (cheddar, mozzarella, or a mix)
- 1/2 cup bell peppers, sliced
- 1/4 cup red onion, sliced
- 1/4 cup spinach, chopped
- 1 tablespoon olive oil

Possible Substitutes:
- Use different vegetables like mushrooms or zucchini
- Add black beans for extra protein

Method of Preparation:
1. Heat olive oil in a skillet over medium heat.
2. Add bell peppers and red onion, cooking until tender.
3. Remove from heat and stir in spinach.
4. Place one tortilla in the skillet and sprinkle with half of the cheese.
5. Spread the vegetable mixture over the cheese, then top with the remaining cheese and the second tortilla.
6. Cook for 2-3 minutes on each side until the tortillas are golden and the cheese is melted.

7. Slice into wedges and serve hot.

Nutritional Value (per serving):
- Calories: 300
- Carbohydrates: 30g
- Protein: 12g
- Fat: 15g
- Fiber: 5g

Cost per Serving:
Approximately $2.50

7. QUICK CHICKEN TACOS

History:
Tacos are a versatile dish with Mexican origins, loved for their simplicity and variety. These quick chicken tacos are easy to prepare and full of flavour.

Ingredients:
- 2 chicken breasts, cooked and shredded
- 8 small corn tortillas
- 1/2 cup salsa
- 1/2 cup shredded lettuce
- 1/4 cup chopped cilantro
- 1/4 cup diced red onion
- 1 lime, cut into wedges

Possible Substitutes:
- Use ground beef or turkey instead of chicken
- Add avocado or sour cream for extra richness

Method of Preparation:
1. Heat tortillas in a dry skillet over medium heat until warm.
2. Divide shredded chicken among the tortillas.
3. Top with salsa, shredded lettuce, cilantro, and red onion.
4. Serve with lime wedges.

Nutritional Value (per serving):
- Calories: 200
- Carbohydrates: 20g

- Protein: 15g
- Fat: 7g
- Fiber: 3g

Cost per Serving:
Approximately $2.00

8. MEDITERRANEAN TUNA SALAD

History:
Mediterranean tuna salad is inspired by the flavours of the Mediterranean diet, known for its health benefits. This salad combines tuna with fresh vegetables and a simple dressing.

Ingredients:
- 1 can (5 oz) tuna, drained

- 1/2 cup cherry tomatoes, halved
- 1/4 cup red onion, finely chopped
- 1/4 cup cucumber, diced
- 1/4 cup Kalamata olives, sliced
- 2 tablespoons olive oil
- 1 tablespoon lemon juice
- 1 teaspoon dried oregano
- Salt and pepper to taste

Possible Substitutes:
- Use salmon or chicken instead of tuna
- Add feta cheese for extra flavour

Method of Preparation:
1. In a large bowl, combine tuna, cherry tomatoes, red onion, cucumber, and olives.
2. In a small bowl, whisk together olive oil, lemon juice, oregano, salt, and pepper.
3. Pour the dressing over the salad and toss to combine.

4. Serve immediately.

Nutritional Value (per serving):
- Calories: 200
- Carbohydrates: 10g
- Protein: 20g
- Fat: 12g
- Fiber: 3g

Cost per Serving:
Approximately $2.50

9. VEGGIE-PACKED MINESTRONE

History:
Minestrone is a traditional Italian soup made with a variety of vegetables and often pasta or rice. This quick version is packed with vegetables and perfect for a nutritious meal.

Ingredients:
- 4 cups vegetable broth
- 1 can (15 oz) diced tomatoes
- 1 cup zucchini, diced
- 1 cup carrots, diced
- 1 cup green beans, cut into pieces
- 1/2 cup pasta (optional)
- 1/2 cup spinach, chopped
- 1/4 cup chopped basil
- 2 cloves garlic, minced
- 1 tablespoon olive oil
- Salt and pepper to taste

Possible Substitutes:
- Use rice or quinoa instead of pasta
- Any preferred vegetables like peas or corn

Method of Preparation:
1. Heat olive oil in a large pot over medium heat.
2. Add garlic, zucchini, carrots, and green beans, cooking until tender.
3. Stir in vegetable broth, diced tomatoes, and pasta (if using).

4. Bring to a boil, then reduce heat and simmer for 15-20 minutes.

5. Stir in spinach and basil, cooking for another 2-3 minutes.

6. Season with salt and pepper.

7. Serve hot.

Nutritional Value (per serving):
- Calories: 150
- Carbohydrates: 25g
- Protein: 5g
- Fat: 4g
- Fiber: 5g

Cost per Serving:
Approximately $2.00

10. INSTANT POT LENTIL CURRY

History:
Lentil curry is a staple in Indian cuisine, known for its rich flavours and hearty texture. Using an Instant Pot makes this dish quick and easy to prepare.

Ingredients:
- 1 cup dried lentils
- 1 can (14.5 oz) diced tomatoes
- 1 onion, diced
- 2 cloves garlic, minced
- 1-inch piece of ginger, grated
- 1 tablespoon curry powder
- 1 teaspoon ground cumin
- 1 teaspoon turmeric
- 2 cups vegetable broth
- 1/2 cup coconut milk
- 1 tablespoon olive oil
- Salt and pepper to taste

Possible Substitutes:
- Use any type of lentils like red or green
- Add vegetables like spinach or bell peppers

Method of Preparation:
1. Set the Instant Pot to sauté mode and heat olive oil.
2. Add onion, garlic, and ginger, cooking until fragrant.
3. Stir in curry powder, cumin, and turmeric.

4. Add lentils, diced tomatoes, vegetable broth, salt, and pepper.
5. Close the lid and set the Instant Pot to manual mode for 15 minutes.
6. Once the cooking is done, release the pressure and stir in coconut milk.
7. Serve hot.

Nutritional Value (per serving):
- Calories: 250
- Carbohydrates: 35g
- Protein: 10g
- Fat: 8g
- Fiber: 12g

Cost per Serving:
Approximately $2.50

EPILOGUE

As we conclude "The Cookbook for Diabetics - 100 Most Popular Tasty and Healthy Dishes from Across the World," we hope you have discovered the immense possibilities that healthy cooking can offer. This book is not just a collection of recipes but a guide to living a healthier, more vibrant life, especially for those managing diabetes.

Throughout these pages, we have explored a myriad of flavours, from the simplicity of a Greek yogurt breakfast to the richness of Moroccan chickpea stew. Each recipe has been carefully selected and crafted to ensure it meets the nutritional needs of diabetics while never compromising on taste or enjoyment. The diversity of dishes reflects the beautiful array of global cuisines, showing that eating healthily can be a culinary adventure rather than a chore.

Embracing a Healthy Lifestyle:
Cooking and eating with diabetes in mind is not just about managing blood sugar levels; it's about embracing a lifestyle that celebrates health and well-being. The recipes provided are tools to help you make better food choices, but they are also meant to inspire creativity in the kitchen. Use them as a foundation and feel free to modify them according to your tastes and preferences. Experiment with different herbs, spices, and ingredients to keep your meals exciting and satisfying.

The Journey of Cooking:
Remember that cooking is a journey, not a destination. There

will be successes and occasional mishaps, but each experience contributes to your growth as a home cook. Cooking should be a joyful and fulfilling activity, a way to nourish both body and soul. Share these meals with family and friends and take pride in the love and care that goes into every dish.

Supporting Each Other:
Managing diabetes can be challenging, but you are not alone. There is a community of individuals who share similar experiences and can offer support, advice, and encouragement. Consider joining local or online groups where you can exchange tips, recipes, and stories. Building a support network can provide invaluable assistance and motivation.

Looking Ahead:
As you move forward, continue to prioritize your health and well-being. Keep exploring new recipes and culinary techniques. Stay informed about the latest nutrition research and how it can benefit your health. Most importantly, listen to your body and consult with healthcare professionals to ensure that your dietary choices align with your health goals.

Final Thoughts:
In closing, we hope this cookbook has not only provided you with delicious recipes but also empowered you with the knowledge and confidence to make healthy cooking an integral part of your life. The journey to managing diabetes through diet is a path to a healthier, happier you.

Thank you for allowing us to be a part of your culinary journey. We wish you health, happiness, and countless delicious meals.

Happy cooking!

"Let food be thy medicine and medicine be thy food."

– Hippocrates

ACKNOWLEDGEMEN TS

I would like to express my deepest gratitude to everyone who has supported the creation of this cookbook. First and foremost, thank you to all the patients and individuals living with diabetes who have inspired this work. Your resilience and determination to lead healthy lives have been a driving force behind this project.

A big thank you to my friend Chinmoyee who first gave the idea of writing this cookbook.

A special thanks to my family and friends for their unwavering support and encouragement throughout this journey. Your feedback, taste-testing, and patience have been invaluable.

To the entire team at Irene Minds & Education, your dedication and hard work have made this book possible. Thank you for believing in this project and helping to bring it to life.

Lastly, I am grateful to the culinary experts, nutritionists, and healthcare professionals whose insights and expertise have enriched the content of this cookbook. Your contributions have ensured that the recipes are delicious, nutritionally balanced, and beneficial for those managing diabetes.

Thank you all for your support and collaboration.

Dr. Bhaskar Bora

COPYRIGHT INFORMATION

LEGAL DISCLAIMER

The information provided in this cookbook is for educational and informational purposes only and is not intended as medical advice. The recipes and dietary suggestions are designed to help individuals manage their diabetes through nutrition, but they should not replace the advice, diagnosis, or treatment of a qualified healthcare professional.

Always consult with your physician or a registered dietitian before making any significant changes to your diet or exercise routine, especially if you have a medical condition. The author and publisher disclaim any liability arising directly or indirectly from the use of this book and assume no responsibility for errors, inaccuracies, or omissions.

The nutritional information provided for each recipe is based on standard calculations and may vary depending on the specific ingredients and brands used. Readers are encouraged to read labels, consider their individual dietary needs, and use their best judgment when preparing and consuming the recipes.

Contact Information:
For inquiries or further information, please contact Dr. Bhaskar Bora at bora.dr@gmail.com